Clinical Practical Record Book of
Psychiatric Nursing

for Undergraduates & Diploma Nursing Students

(As per the Revised INC Syllabus)

● **Third Edition** ●

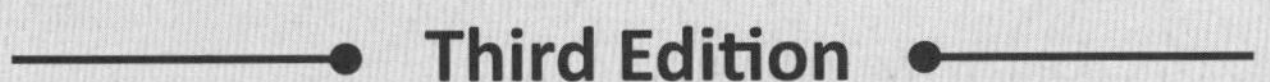

Kallappa M Sollapure MSc Nursing (Psychiatric Nursing)
Assistant Professor
Shri JG Co-operative Hospital Society's
Institute of Nursing, Ghataprabha, Karnataka

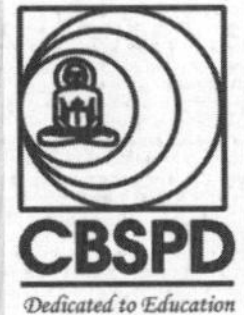

CBS Publishers and Distributors Pvt Ltd

• New Delhi • Bengaluru • Chennai • Kochi • Kolkata • Lucknow • Mumbai
• Hyderabad • Jharkhand • Nagpur • Patna • Pune • Uttarakhand

Clinical
Practical Record Book of

Psychiatric Nursing

for Undergraduates & Diploma Nursing Students

(As per the Revised INC Syllabus)

ISBN: 978-93-94525-79-5

Copyright © Author and Publishers

Reprint: 2026

Third Edition: 2025

Second Edition: 2019

Published by **Satish Kumar Jain** and produced by **Varun Jain** for

CBS Publishers and Distributors Pvt Ltd

4819/XI Prahlad Street, 24 Ansari Road, Daryaganj, New Delhi 110 002, India.
Ph: 23289259, 23266861, 23266867   Website: www.cbspd.com
Fax: 011-23243014
e-mail: delhi@cbspd.com; cbspubs@airtelmail.in.
Corporate Office: 204 FIE, Industrial Area, Patparganj, Delhi 110 092
Ph: 4934 4934   Fax: 4934 4935
e-mail: feedback@cbspd.com; bhupesharora@cbspd.com

Branches

- **Bengaluru:** Seema House 2975, 17th Cross, K.R. Road, Banashankari 2nd Stage, Bengaluru-560 070, Karnataka
  Ph: +91-80-26771678/79   Fax: +91-80-26771680   e-mail: bangalore@cbspd.com
- **Chennai:** 7, Subbaraya Street, Shenoy Nagar, Chennai-600 030, Tamil Nadu
  Ph: +91-44-26680620, 26681266   Fax: +91-44-42032115   e-mail: chennai@cbspd.com
- **Kochi:** 68/1534, 35, 36-Power House Road, Opp. KSEB, Cochin-682018, Kochi, Kerala
  Ph: +91-484-4059061-65   Fax: +91-484-4059065   e-mail: kochi@cbspd.com
- **Kolkata:** Hind Ceramics Compound, 1st Floor, 147, Nilganj Road, Belghoria, Kolkata-700056, West Bengal
  Ph: +91-033-2563-3055/56   e-mail: kolkata@cbspd.com
- **Lucknow:** Basement, Khushnuma Complex, 7-Meerabai Marg (Behind Jawahar Bhawan), Lucknow-226001, Uttar Pradesh
  Ph: +0522-4000032   e-mail: tiwari.lucknow@cbspd.com
- **Mumbai:** PWD Shed, Gala No. 25/26, Ramchandra Bhatt Marg, Next to J.J. Hospital Gate No. 2, Opp. Union Bank of India, Noor Baug, Mumbai-400009, Maharashtra
  Ph: +91-22-66661880/89   Fax: +91-22-24902342   e-mail: mumbai@cbspd.com

Representatives

- **Hyderabad** +91-9885175004
- **Jharkhand** +91-9811541605
- **Nagpur** +91-9421945513
- **Patna** +91-9334159340
- **Pune** +91-9623451994
- **Uttarakhand** +91-9716462459

Printed at : Goyal Offset Works Pvt. Ltd. Haryana

Preface

Psychiatric Nursing or Mental Health Nursing is an essential aspect of healthcare system. Hence, this subject has been included in nursing curriculum as one of the major subjects in India and abroad as well.

The Indian Nursing Council has prescribed compulsory psychiatric clinical training for both Diploma and BSc Nursing students. To help the students to fulfill clinical requirements in mental health subject, this practical record book has been prepared.

Utmost care has been taken to make this record book handy and student friendly. Contents are organized to meet the requirements prescribed by the nursing curriculum. This book is meant for both Diploma and BSc Nursing students.

The purpose of this record book is to provide guidelines to the students to complete clinical requirements as well as to help them systematically organize their learning in the psychiatric clinical setting. The seniors, colleagues and students' opinion and guidelines have been followed to finalize the overall content of the book.

Last but not least, I extend my special thanks to **Mr Satish Kumar Jain** (Chairman) and **Mr Varun Jain** (Managing Director), M/s CBS Publishers and Distributors Pvt Ltd for their wholehearted support in publication of this book. I have no words to describe the role, efforts, inputs and initiatives undertaken by **Mr Bhupesh Aarora** [Sr. Vice President – Publishing & Marketing (Health Sciences Division)] for helping and motivating me.

I sincerely thank the entire CBS team for bringing out the book with utmost care and attractive presentation. I would like to thank Ms Nitasha Arora (Assistant General Manager Publishing – Medical and Nursing), and Dr Anju Dhir (Sr. Product Manager and Medical Development Editor) for their publishing support. I would also extend my thanks to Ms Surbhi Gupta, Team Lead (Editorial), Mr Ashutosh Pathak (Assistant Production Manager) and all the production team members for devoting laborious hours in editing, designing and typesetting the book.

Kallappa M Sollapure

Name of the Institution

CERTIFICATE
Department of Mental Health Nursing

This is to certify that Mr/Ms ____ with Registration no. _________________ has satisfactorily completed his/her requirements of Mental Health Nursing as prescribed by **Indian Nursing Council, New Delhi**, and __

____

University/Board during the year _______________.

Date:

Place:

Signature of Subject Incharge   **Signature of HOD**

Signature of Principal

Internal Examiner   **External Examiner**

1. _____________________   1. _____________________

2. _____________________   2. _____________________

3. _____________________   3. _____________________

Requirements

Diploma in Nursing

Sl. no.	Requirements	Number of forms
1.	History taking	2
2.	Mental status examination	2
3.	Process recording	2
4.	Care plan	1
5.	Case study	1
6.	Case presentation	1
7.	OPD visit report	1
8.	Visit to child guidance clinic	1
9.	Health education	2
10.	Drug book (10 drugs)	10
11.	Attending and assisting various therapies	5

Basic BSc and Post Basic BSc in Nursing

Sl. no.	Requirements	Number of forms
1.	History taking	5
2.	Mental status examination	5
3.	Mini mental status examination	2
4.	Process recording/verbatim	2
5.	Care plan	5
6.	Case study	3
7.	Case presentation	2
8.	Visit report	2
9.	Health education	2
10.	Drug book (10 drugs)	10
11.	Attending and assisting various therapies	5

Contents

Area	Sl. no.	Contents	Page no.	Date	Signature of the supervisor
Therapies	31.	Assignment on Psychotherapies	185		
	32.	1.			
	33.	2.			
	34.	3.			
	35.	4.			
	36.	5.			
	37.	Drug Study (10 Drugs)	200		
	38.	Health Education—Individual	220		
	39.	Health Education—Group	225		
De-addiction centre	40.	Psychiatric Care Study on Drug Dependency	231		
	41.	Observation Report on Visit to De-addiction Center	247		
	42.	Observation Report on Visit to Rehabilitation Center	250		

Name and Signature of Subject in charge

Name and Signature HOD

MENTAL HEALTH

Mental health is an important aspect of health. As per World Health Organization (WHO), **'health is a state of complete physical, mental, social and spiritual well-being, not merely the absence of disease or infirmity'.** This indicates that any individual to be called healthy he must be in a state of complete well-being, i.e., physically, mentally, socially and spiritually.

Definition of Mental Health

"There is no single precise definition for mental health. In general, mental health can be viewed as a state of well-being in which an individual realizes his/her own abilities, can cope with the normal stresses of life, can work productively and fruitfully and can to make a contribution to his/her community".

According to American Psychiatric Association (APA)

"Mental health is a simultaneous success at working, loving and creating with the capacity for mature and flexible resolution of conflicts between instincts, conscience, important other people and reality".

Characteristics of Mentally Healthy Individual

The Mentally Healthy Individuals

- Are not overwhelmed by their emotions like fear, anger, love, jealousy, guilt or worries.
- Know their own strengths and weakness
- Have self-respect
- Deal with most situations independently
- Accept their own shortcomings
- Can give love and considerations to others
- Keep satisfying and long-lasting personal relationships
- Can develop trust in others
- Respect others rights and feelings
- Can feel as part of the groups
- Accept the roles and responsibilities in family, work and society
- Can adjust with their environmental changes or modify environment wherever possible
- Keep realistic goal or dream
- Enjoy happiness with their loved ones and share their worries with their closed ones.

MENTAL ILLNESS

A universal definition of mental illness is difficult because various factors like culture influence the definition of mental illness. In general, mental illness is maladjustment in living. The mental illness is disharmony between the individual and his/her surroundings.

Society also defines mental illness. Individual will be labeled as mentally ill if his/her behavior is not culturally defined by that society. That's how one individual who is considered mentally healthy may be viewed as mentally ill in another society, as the normal and abnormal behaviors are culturally defined.

According to WHO

"Mental and behavioral disorders are understood as clinically significant conditions characterized by alterations in thinking, mood or behavior associated with personal distress and/or impaired functioning".

According to American Psychiatric Association (2000)

"Mental illness is a clinically significant behavioral or psychological syndrome or pattern that occurs in a person and that is associated with present distress or disability or with a significantly increased risk of suffering death, pain, disability or an important loss of freedom… and is not merely an expectable and culturally sanctioned response to a particular event".

Characteristics of Mental Illness

- Change in one's thinking, memory, perception, emotion and judgment resulting in change in speech and behavior which is deviant from his/her previous personality.
- Change in behavior causes distress and suffering to the individual or others or to the both.
- Changes in behavior and distress lead to disturbances in the daily activities, occupation and relationship with important others.

ICD 10 (INTERNATIONAL CLASSIFICATION OF DISEASE AND RELATED HEALTH PROBLEMS)–1990

ICD 10 is WHO's classification for all diseases and related health problems. WHO has classified all the diseases and health-related-problems based on alphanumerical system. Mental disorders were not included in the international classification until its 6th edition (1948). The 8th edition of ICD (1965) made some progress toward solving the earlier problems but it was still unsatisfactory. The improvements were made in 9th edition.

Present 10th edition of ICD (1990) has got special chapter for mental and behavioral disorders. The chapter 'F' classifies psychiatric disorders as mental and behavioral disorders and codes them on an alphanumeric system from **F00 to F99.**

SUMMARY OF CLASSIFICATION OF PSYCHIATRIC DISORDERS BY WHO IN ICD 10

Organic, Including Symptomatic Mental Disorders (F00–F09)

F00–Dementia in Alzheimer's disease

F01–Vascular dementia

F02–Dementia in other diseases classified elsewhere

F03–Unspecified dementia

F04–Organic amnestic syndrome

F05–Delirium, not induced by alcohol and other psychoactive substances

F06–Other mental disorders due to brain damage and dysfunction and physical disease

F07–Personality and behavioral disorders due to brain disease, damage and dysfunction

F09–unspecified organic or symptomatic mental disorder

Mental and Behavioral Disorders Due to Psychoactive Substance Use (F10–19)

F10–Mental and behavioral disorders due to use of alcohol

F11–Mental and behavioral disorders due to use of opioids

F12–Mental and behavioral disorders due to use of cannabinoids

F13–Mental and behavioral disorders due to use of sedatives and hypnotics

F14–Mental and behavioral disorders due to use of cocaine

F15–Mental and behavioral disorders due to use of other stimulants, including caffeine

F16–Mental and behavioral disorders due to use of hallucinogens

F17–Mental and behavioral disorders due to use of tobacco

F18–Mental and behavioral disorders due to use of volatile solvent

F19–Mental and behavioral disorders due to multiple drug use and use of other psychoactive substances

Schizophrenia, Schizotypal and Delusional Disorders (F20–29)

F20–Schizophrenia

F21–Schizotypal disorder

F22–Persistent delusional disorders

F23–Acute and Transient psychotic disorders

F24–Induced Delusional disorders

F25–Schizoaffective disorders

F28–Other nonorganic psychotic disorders

F29–Unspecified nonorganic psychosis

Mood (Affective) Disorders (F30–39)

F30–Manic episode

F31–Bipolar affective disorder

F32–Depressive episode

F33–Recurrent depressive disorder

F34–Persistent mood disorder

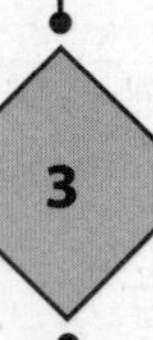

F35–Other mood (affective) disorders

F39–Unspecified mood (affective) disorders

Neurotic, Stress Related and Somatoform Disorders (F40–49)

F40–Phobic anxiety disorders

F41–Other anxiety disorders

F42–Obsessive-compulsive disorder

F43–Reaction to severe stress and adjustment disorders

F44–Dissociative (Conversion) disorders

F45–Somatoform disorders

F48–Other neurotic disorders

Behavioral Syndromes Associated with Physiological Disturbances and Physical Factors (F50–59)

F50–Eating Disorders

F51–Nonorganic sleep disorders

F52–Sexual dysfunction not caused by organic disorders

F53–Mental and behavioral disorders associated with puerperium, not elsewhere classified

Disorders of Adult Personality Behavior (F60–69)

F60–Specific personality disorders

F61–Mixed and other personality disorders

F62–Enduring personality changes, not attributable to brain damage and disease

F63–Habit and impulse disorders

F64–Gender identity disorders

F65–Disorders of sexual preference

Mental Retardation (F70–79)

F70–Mild Mental Retardation

F71–Moderate Mental Retardation

F72–Severe Mental Retardation

F73–Profound Mental Retardation

F78–Other mental retardation

F79–Unspecified mental retardation

Disorders of Psychological Development (F80–89)

F80–Specific developmental disorders of speech and language

F81–Specific developmental disorders of scholastic skills

F82–Specific developmental disorders of motor function

F83–Mixed specific developmental disorders

F84–Pervasive developmental disorders

F88–Other psychological developmental disorders

F89–Unspecified psychological developmental disorders

Behavioral and Emotional Disorders with Onset Usually Occurring in Childhood and Adolescence (F90-98)

F90–Hyperkinetic disorders

F91–Conduct disorders

F93–Emotional disorders with onset specific to childhood

F94–Disorders of social functioning with onset specific to childhood and adolescence

F95–Tic Disorders

F98–Other behavioral and emotional disorders with onset usually occurring in childhood and adolescence

Unspecified mental Disorders (F99)

F99–Mental disorder not otherwise specified

MENTAL HEALTH NURSING

Human being is a social animal. People come across various stressors, which at a time are overwhelming when living in complex society. Everyone experiences some degree of loss, despair and confusion in day-to-day life. Some of these experiences become too hard to overcome from them. When individuals fail to overcome these experiences effectively in an adaptive way they may get into behavioral disturbances which puts them in need of professional help to overcome. In such situations mental health professionals play their role in helping the needy individuals.

The mental health nursing professionals deal with the factors related to illness and work for the promotion of mental health of the mentally ill.

Definitions

- *"Mental health nursing is a specialized area of nursing practice directed toward the prevention, treatment and rehabilitative aspects of mental health care."*
- ***According to APA,*** *"Mental health nursing is specialized area of nursing practice, combination of science and art by employing theories of human behavior applied in the diagnosis and treatment of human response to actual or potential mental health problems. It deals with promotion of mental health, prevention of mental illness, care of the client with mental illness, cure of mental illness and rehabilitation of mentally ill patients in the hospital and community".*

Psychiatric Assessment

Nursing assessment is done to elicit information from patients to identify problems and to formulate plans for interventions.

Purposes of Psychiatric Assessment are

- To allow the client and his relatives to express their feelings in their own words
- To describe the patient's condition
- To explore the family, developmental and environmental factors affecting his behavior.
- To find out the predisposing causes and primary causes of his behavior
- To make identify needs and problems of the patient and to make appropriate nursing diagnosis
- To plan and implement appropriate nursing interventions.

Psychiatric Assessment Includes the Following

- Psychiatric history collection
- Mental status examination
- Physical examination
- Biological investigations
- Psychological investigation

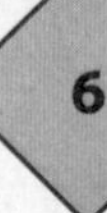

Psychiatric History Collection

Psychiatric history collection is the first step in psychiatric assessment. It includes identification of patient's personal data and collection of detailed information about patient's present and past illness along with his/her personal and family history. The history collection is done under the following headings:

- Demographic/identification data
- Presenting chief complaints
- History of present illness
- Past health history
- Family health history
- Personal history

Steps for Taking Psychiatric History

- **Identification of data**
- **Informant**
  - Relationship with the patient
  - Intimacy with the patient
  - Does the informant live with the patient?
  - Duration of relationship with the patient
  - Bias with the patient
  - Interest of the informant in the patient's property or money
- **Presenting complaints or problems**

  As experienced by the patient: A clear statement of problems and complaints should be obtained from the patient if possible, record "VERBATIM" (word for word what the patient says). As described by the patient's relative(s):

  Information from the patient's relative should be collected for getting complete history.

- **History of present illness**

  Give a detailed and coherent account of the symptoms from the onset to the time of consultation including their chronological evolution and course. Specific attention must be paid to the following:

  Onset: Note the onset of symptoms is abrupt (within 48 hours), acute (developing within few days to 2 weeks), subacute (few weeks), or insidious (few weeks to few months)

  Precipitating factors: Enquire about any precipitating events. These could be physical (e.g., febrile illness) or psychological in nature (loss/death). Ascertain whether events clearly preceded the illness or were consequences of illness.

  Course of the illness: The course of illness can be episodic, or fluctuating. In addition, a different pattern of symptoms may evolve in a continuous illness.

  Associated disturbances: Enquiry should be made about impairment in other areas of functioning. These include sleep, appetite, weight, sexual life, social life and occupation. The specific nature of the disturbance and degree of disability should be recorded.

- **Personal history:**
  - **Birth and early development:** Record the prenatal, natal and postnatal periods, was the birth at full term? Whether delivered in hospital or at home? Any complications during delivery? Any physical illnesses in the post-natal period? Ascertain whether milestones of development were normal or delayed.

- **Childhood:** Enquire about sleep disturbance, thumb-sucking, nail-biting, temper tantrum, bed wetting, stammering, tics, and mannerism. Look out for conduct disturbances in the form of frequent fights, truancy, stealing, lying and gang activities. Also enquire about relationship with parents, sibling and peers.

- **Physical illness during childhood:** Record physical illness suffered in childhood. Enquire specifically regarding epilepsy, meningitis and encephalitis.

- **Educational history:** Enquire also about age of beginning and finishing school, type of school attended. Scholastic performance, attitudes toward peers and teachers. Any school phobia, non-attendance, truancy, any learning difficulties and reason for termination of studies

- **Play history:** The questions to be asked are, what games were played at what stage, with whom and where. Relationship with peers, particularly the opposite sex, should be recorded.

- **Puberty:** The age at menarche and reaction to menarche (in females), the age at appearance of secondary sexual characteristics, nocturnal emission (in males), masturbation and any anxiety related to puberty changes to be asked.

- **Menstrual and obstetric history:** The regularity of menses, the length of each cycle, any abnormalities, the last menstrual period, the number of children born, termination of pregnancy, if any, should be asked for.

- **Occupational history:** The age at starting work; jobs held in chronological order; reasons for changes; job satisfaction; ambitions; relationships with authorities, peers, and subordinates; present income; and whether the job is appropriate to the educational and family background should be asked.

- **Sexual and marital history:** Sexual information, how acquired and what kind; masturbation (fantasy and activity); sex play, if any; adolescent sexual activity; premarital and extramarital relationships, if any; sexual practices (normal and abnormal); and any gender identity disorder, are the areas to be inquired about.

- The duration of marriage; the time spent knowing partner before marriage, marriage arranged by parents or without the consent of parents, number of marriages, divorce or separation, role in marriage, interpersonal and sexual relationship, contraceptives used, sexual satisfaction and frequency of intercourse; and psychosexual dysfunction should be asked.

- **Pre-morbid personality:** It is important to elicit details regarding the personality of individual.

  - **Interpersonal Relationship:** Interpersonal relationship with family members, friends, work-mates and superiors; introverted/extroverted; ease of making and keeping social relations.
  - **Use of leisure time:** Hobbies; interests; intellectual activities; critical faculty; energetic/sedentary.
  - **Predominant mood:** Optimistic/pessimistic; stable/prone to anxiety; cheerful/despondent; reaction to stressful life events.
  - **Attitude to self or others:** Self-confidence level; self-criticism; self-consciousness; selfish/thoughtful of others; self-appraisal of abilities, achievements or failures.
  - **Attitude to work and responsibility:** Decision making; acceptance of responsibility; flexibility; perseverance; foresight.
  - **Religious beliefs and moral attitudes:** Religious beliefs; tolerance of others' standards and beliefs; conscience; altruism.
  - **Fantasy life:** Sexual and nonsexual fantasies; daydreaming- frequency and content; recurrent or favorite daydreams; dreams.
  - **Habits:** Food fads; alcohol; tobacco; drugs; sleep.

Mental Status Examination

Mental status examination (MSE) is the structured way of observing and describing a patient's current state of mind, under the domains of appearance, behavior, mood, affect, speech, thought process, thought content, perception, cognition and insight.

The purpose of MSE is to obtain a comprehensive description of patient's mental state. Along with psychiatric history, MSE helps to make accurate clinical diagnosis of patient's condition.

DOMAINS OF MSE ("ASEPTIC")

A - Appearance/behavior and psychomotor activity

S - Speech

E - Emotion (mood and affect)

P - Perception (auditory/visual hallucinations)

T - Thought content (suicidal/homicidal ideation) and Process

I - Insight and judgment

C - Cognition

Appearance and Behavior:	The appearance of the patient may provide some clues regarding their lifestyle, current mental state and ability to care for themselves. • Apparent age • Height and Weight • Manner of dress and grooming • Hygiene • Hair color and texture • Evidence of scars, tattoos, signs of intravenous drug use or other skin marks • Any odor
Behavior:	A patient's behavior may provide insights into his/her current mental state. • Engagement and rapport • Eye contact • Facial expression • Body language
Psychomotor activity:	Observe any evidence of psychomotor abnormalities: • Psychomotor retardation • Increased Restlessness • Abnormal movements or postures
Speech:	The patient's speech is assessed by observing his/her spontaneous speech, and also by using structured tests of specific language functions. • Initiation • Rate of speech • Quantity of speech • Tone of speech • Volume of speech • Fluency and rhythm of speech
Emotion (Mood and affect):	Mood and affect both relate to emotion, however, they are fundamentally different. Affect represents immediately expressed and observed emotion (e.g., the patient's facial expression or overall demeanor). Affect is what you observe. Mood represents a patient's predominant subjective internal state at any one time as described by them. Mood is what the patient tells you. • Mood state (Predominant emotion over days/weeks) • Apparent affect (Current observed emotional state) • Range and mobility of affect • Intensity of affect • Congruency of affect
Perception	Perception involves the organization, identification and interpretation of sensory information to understand the world around us. Abnormalities of perception signify several mental health conditions. • Altered Bodily Experiences (Depersonalization/Derealization) • Hallucinations/Illusions
Thought process:	• Thought process in the MSE refers to the quantity, tempo (rate of flow) and form (or logical coherence) of thought. Thought process cannot be directly observed but can only be described by the patient or inferred from a patient's speech. • Thought can be described in terms of form, content and possession.
Thought form:	• Thought stream (Speed and flow), Poverty of thought (thought blocking), poverty of content (perseveration), racing thoughts, flight of ideas. • Logical and goal directed thought directed A→B (normal) v/s formal thought disorders such as loose associations/Circumstantial thoughts/Tangential thoughts/Flight of ideas/Thought blocking/Perseveration/Neologisms • Thought content: Delusions/ Obsessions/Compulsions/Phobias/Overvalued ideas/Suicidal thoughts / Homicidal/Violent thoughts • Thought possession: Thought insertion/Thought withdrawal/Thought broadcasting

Contd...

Insight and judgment:	Insight, in a mental state examination context, refers to the ability of a patient to understand that he/she has a mental health problem and that what he/she is experiencing is abnormal. **Insight can be described as:** • Poor (patient may be in complete denial of their symptoms or diagnosis, or there may be slight awareness) • Fair (The patient may understand their symptoms or diagnosis intellectual "on paper," but fail to understand it emotionally, or fully grasp the impact of it on his/her life) • Good/Excellent (Overall, a good intellectual and emotional understanding of his/her symptoms or difficulties. Patient is acutely aware of symptoms or illness, and also of their own limitations and strengths. Symptoms are likely to be in remission, and the patient knows when to reach out for help and when to rely on himself/herself.) Judgment refers to the ability to make considered decisions or come to a sensible conclusion when presented with information.
Cognition:	Cognition refers to "the mental action or process of acquiring knowledge and understanding through thought, experience, and the senses". Cognition can be impaired as a result of mental health conditions and their treatments. This section of the MSE covers the patient's level of alertness, orientation, attention, memory, visuospatial functioning, language functions and executive functions. • Level of alertness • **Orientation:** Time/Place/Person • Attention • Concentration • **Memory:** Immediate/Recent/Remote • **Visuospatial functioning:** (can be assessed by the ability to copy a diagram, draw a clock face, or draw a map of the consulting room.) • Language (is assessed through the ability to name objects, repeat phrases, and by observing the individual's spontaneous speech and response to instructions.) • Executive functioning (can be screened for by asking the "similarities" questions ("what do x and y have in common?") and by means of a verbal fluency task (e.g., "list as many words as you can start with the letter F, in one minute").

Physical Examination

The aim is to exclude:
- Physical causes of psychiatric symptoms
- Coexistent physical disorder
- Physical consequences of psychiatric disorder

Biological Investigations

Investigations include the following:
- General medical screening
- **Toxicology screen:** Useful when substance use is suspected, e.g., alcohol, cocaine, opiates, cannabis, phencyclidine, benzodiazepines, barbiturates.
- **Drug levels:** Drug levels are indicated to test for therapeutic blood levels, for toxic blood levels and for testing drug compliance. For example, lithium (0.6–1.6 mEq/L), haloperidol (8–18 ng/mL), valproate (50–100 µg/mL).

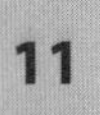

- **Electrophysiological tests**
  - Electroencephalogram (EEG)
  - Brain electrical activity mapping (BEAM)
  - Video telemetry EEG
  - Polysomnography
  - Holter EKG
- **Brain imaging tests**
  - **Computed tomography scan**: Dementia, delirium, seizures,
  - **Magnetic resonance imaging**: Dementia, higher resolution than CT scan
  - **Positron emission test (PET)**: For study of brain functioning and physiology
  - **Single positron emission computed tomography (SPECT)**: Research tool
  - **Magnetic resonance angiography**
- **Neuroendocrine tests**
  - **Dexamethasone suppression test (DST):** Research tool in depression (response to antidepressants or ECT)
  - **TRH stimulation test:** Lithium-induced hypothyroidism, refractory depression. If the serum TSH is >35 µIU/mL (following 500 mg of TRH given IV), the test is positive.
  - **Serum prolactin levels:** Seizures versus pseudoseizures, galactorrhea with antipsychotics.
  - **Serum 17 hydroxycorticosteroid:** Organic mood disorders
- **Biochemical tests:**
  - **5- HIAA:** Research tool (depression, suicidal and/or aggressive behavior)
  - **MHPG:** Research tool (depression)
  - **Catecholamine levels:** Organic anxiety disorders
- **Genetics tests:** Cytogenetic workup is useful in some cases of mental retardation.
- **Sexual disorder investigation:**
  - **Papaverine test**: Male erectile disorder (intracavernosal injection of papaverine is sometimes used to differentiate organic from nonorganic male erectile disorder)
  - Serum Testosterone
  - Penile Doppler: Male erectile disorder.

Psychological Investigations

- **Objective tests:** These are pen and paper, objective tests, which are employed to test various aspects of personality and intelligence in a person.
- **Projective tests:** In projective tests, ambiguous stimuli are used which are not clear to the person immediately. For example, Sentence completion tests, thematic apperception test, Draw-a-person test (DAPT).
- **Neuropsychological tests:** Some of the commonly used neuropsychological tests are Wisconsin card sorting test, Wechsler memory scale, PGI memory scale, Bender Gestalt test, etc.
- **Rating scales:** Several rating scales are used in psychiatry to quantify the psychopathology observed. Some of the commonly used scales are Brief psychiatric rating scales (BPRS), Scale for assessment of negative symptoms (SANS) and Scale for assessment of positive symptoms (SAPS).

Mini-Mental Status Examination

The **mini-mental state examination** (**MMSE**) is a brief 30-point questionnaire test that is used to screen for cognitive impairment. It is commonly used in medicine to screen for dementia. It is also used to estimate the severity of cognitive impairment at a given point in time and to follow the course of cognitive changes in an individual over time, thus making it an effective way to document an individual's response to treatment.

This test is not the same thing as a mental status examination. In the time span of about 10 minutes, it examines various functions including arithmetic, memory and orientation. It was introduced by Folstein *et. al.* in 1975.

Process Recording

Process recording is a way of evaluating patient's condition and assessing his/her behavior. It is an exact written record of conversation and actions between the nurse and patient during the time they are together. It also records nurse's feeling about what was going on at the time and observation of the patient's behavior during the conversation.

The interaction or interview is recorded by the nurse by using various communication skills. During conversation nurse draws interference. Recording of the interview is called a process recording.

Purposes of Process Recording

- Assists the nurse or student to plan, structure and evaluate the interaction on a conscious rather than intuitive level.
- Assists the nurse to gain competency in interpreting and synthesizing raw data under supervision.
- Helps to consciously apply theory to practice.
- Helps the nurse to develop an increased awareness of behavior, verbal and nonverbal communication patterns and the effect of those patterns on others.
- Helps nurse to learn to identify thoughts and feelings in relation to self or others.
- Helps to increase observational skills.
- Helps to increase ability to identify problems and gain skills to solve those problems.

Steps in Process Recording

- **Collection of raw data:** Raw data includes verbal and nonverbal communication between the nurse and patient.
- **Interpretation:** After going through the data, the nurse interprets the data and analyzes why the behavior was as it was, that is, subject analyzing and level of interpretation.
- **Application of concepts to the data:** Concepts not only explain and predict behavior but also indicate nurse's behavior.
- **Analysis:** Detailed critical assessment of nature and significance of data.
- **Synthesis:** Process of putting analyzed data together to form a unitary whole.

Verbatim/Process Recording Format

Name of patient   : ....

Place   : ....

Date and time   : ....

Situation   : ....

D.O.A   : ....

Objectives of Interview

1. ....
2. ....
3. ....

Verbatim

Person	Verbatim	Nonverbal communication	Inference
Nurse			
Patient			

Conclusion

Summary

- List of inferences
- Care plan made
- Special difficulties faced
- Techniques used to overcome

ELECTROCONVULSIVE THERAPY

Introduction

- Electroconvulsive therapy (ECT) is a physical therapy in which with the help of electrodes, electrical current is passed to the brain to produce generalized seizures.
- Modified electroconvulsive therapy (ECT) is a controlled medical procedure in which a seizure is induced in an anesthetized patient to produce a therapeutic effect.
- ECT is a highly technical procedure requiring a team that consists of an anesthetist, a psychiatrist, psychiatric nurses, and recovery nurses.
- Psychiatric nurses have an important role in caring patients who receive ECT.

Types of ECT

- **Direct ECT:** ECT is administered without anesthesia and muscle relaxant.
- **Modified ECT:** ECT is administered with anesthesia and muscle relaxant.

Application of Electrodes

Electrode is placed at 1–1.5 inch above the midline drawn between outer canthus of eye and tragus muscle of the ear.
- **Unilateral placement:** In unilateral ECT, electrode is placed usually on nondominant side of the brain.
- **Bilateral placement:** In bilateral ECT, electrodes are placed on both the sides.

Amount and Duration of Electric Current Used

As per APA guidelines, 70–120 volts of electric current is used for duration of 0.7–1.5 seconds.

Type of Seizures Produced

Grand Mal Seizure

Tonic phase lasts for 10–15 seconds.
Clonic phase lasts for 30–60 seconds.

Indications for ECT

- Severe depression
- Acute mania
- Mood disorders with psychotic features
- Intolerance to side effects of medication or other treatments.

- Deterioration in condition, or appearance of suicidality or pronounced lethargy.
- Acute catatonia

Contraindications

- Increased intracranial pressure
- Cerebral aneurysm
- Cerebral hemorrhage
- H/o cardiovascular diseases
- Brain tumor
- Acute myocardial infarction
- Congestive heart failure
- Pneumonia
- Aortic aneurysm

Nursing Care in ECT

ECT is treated like a minor surgical procedure that requires preoperative preparation and postoperative care. There are four components of nursing care in ECT:

1. Providing educational and emotional support
2. Pretreatment nursing care
3. Nursing care during procedure
4. Post ECT care

Providing Educational and Emotional Support

- Explain the procedure to the patient.
- Obtain an informed consent from the patient and the carer.
- Respond to patient's concerns and feelings.
- Educate the patient concerning the procedure and explain the necessary tasks associated with ECT to the patient.
- Initiate education interventions based on knowledge deficits.

Pretreatment Nursing Care

- Preparation of treatment suite for the ECT procedure.
- An adjustable height stretcher trolley.
- Complete the pretreatment check list.
- The patient's identity is checked and the patient wears an identity bracelet.
- Ensure safekeeping of the patient's valuables.
- NPO for minimum 4 hours before treatment to prevent possible aspiration during anesthesia.
- The patient's hair should be clean and dry to allow for electrode contact.
- Hairpins, bracelets, body piercing should be removed to avoid burns.
- The patient should be encouraged to pass urine before the treatment to avoid incontinence during the procedure.
- Prostheses, dentures, glasses, hearing aids, contact lenses should be removed.

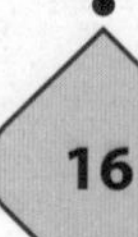

- Minimize anxiety through anxiety management techniques, ensuring short waiting time and offering reassurance and support.
- Standard practices should be adopted regarding general anesthesia care.

Nursing Care during ECT Procedure

- Transfer the patient on a trolley from the waiting room to the ECT room on a well-padded bed and placed in a comfortable dorsal position or supine position. A small pillow is placed under the lumber curve.
- Apply ECG electrodes, BP cuff, and pulse oximetry sensor (not on same extremity as BP cuff).
- Give a short-acting anesthetic agent. Thiopental 0.25 mg to 0.5 mg, IV and scoline (Succinylcholine) 30–50 mg. The dose of drug may vary from patient to patient.
- Prepare EEG electrodes, as per treatment specifications.
- Prepare scalp and stimulus ECT electrodes (unilateral versus bilateral) and apply paste to electrodes.
- Support the shoulder and arms of the patient. Restraint the thigh with the help of a sheet.
- Hyperextension of the head with support to the chin.
- Administer oxygen
- Apply jelly to the electrodes
- Make the observations of the convulsions.
- The presence of initial tonic stage which lasts for 10–15 seconds followed by clonic stage which lasts for 30–60 seconds then there is a phase of muscular relaxation with stertorous respiration, i.e., flaccid stage.
- Do suction immediately
- Restore respiration by giving O_2, if necessary.

Post-ECT Care

- Observe and record the vital parameters
- Place the patient on side lying position, clean the secretions
- Transfer the practient from recovery room. Record vital signs every 15 minutes for 30 minutes and once in every 30 minutes till the patient recovers to the normal stage.
- Allow the patient to sleep for 30 minutes to one hour
- Reassure the patient and reorient to the ward
- Allow the patient to have tea or any drinks
- Record the procedure

Equipment for ECT

- Treatment devices and supplies, including electrode paste and gel, gauze pads, saline, electro encephalogram electrodes and chart paper.
- Monitoring equipment including ECG and EEG electrodes
- BP cuffs, peripheral nerve stimulator and pulse oximeter
- Stethoscope
- Reflex hammer
- Intravenous and venipuncture supplies
- Stretchers with firm mattress with side rails with the capacity of raising the head and foot end
- Bite blocks

- Suction device
- Ventilation equipment, including tubing, masks, Ambu bag, oral airways, intubation equipment with an oxygen delivery system capable of providing positive- pressure oxygen
- Emergency and other medications as recommended by the anesthesia staff
- Miscellaneous medications not supplied by anesthesia staff for medical management during ECT such as midazolam, diazepam, thiopental sodium, glycopyrrolate, succinylcholine, etc.

Documentation

- Document using flow sheets or progress notes.
- Record the patient's vital signs and responses during the treatment sequence, recovery, and post-recovery.
- Document medications, stimulus parameter, seizure response and vital signs
- Assess and document the patient's physical and mental status and any behavioral changes or lack of such changes

Some NANDA Nursing Diagnoses Related Mental and Behavioral Disorders

- Altered sensory perception
- Loss of hope
- Mourning [grief] dysfunctional
- Mourning [grief] in advance
- Post-traumatic reaction
- Self-care, deficit: dressing/grooming
- Recreation, deficit
- Insomnia
- Sleep deprivation
- Readiness for enhanced sleep
- Disturbed sleep pattern
- Self-neglect
- Acute confusion
- Risk of acute confusion
- Chronic confusion
- Labile emotional control
- Ineffective impulse control
- Deficient knowledge
- Readiness for enhanced knowledge
- Impaired memory
- Readiness for enhanced communication
- Impaired verbal communication
- Hopelessness
- Readiness for enhanced hope
- Risk of compromised human dignity
- Disturbed personal identity
- Risk of disturbed personal identity
- Readiness for enhanced self-concept
- Chronic low self-esteem
- Risk of chronic low self-esteem
- Situational low self-esteem
- Risk of situational low self-esteem
- Disturbed body image
- Risk of impaired attachment
- Dysfunctional family processes
- Interrupted family processes
- Readiness for enhanced family processes
- Ineffective relationship
- Risk of ineffective relationship
- Readiness for enhanced relationship
- Ineffective activity planning
- Risk of ineffective activity planning
- Anxiety
- Defensive coping
- Ineffective coping
- Readiness for enhanced coping
- Ineffective community coping
- Readiness for enhanced community coping
- Compromised family coping
- Disabled family coping
- Readiness for enhanced family coping
- Death anxiety
- Ineffective denial
- Fear
- Grieving
- Complicated grieving
- Risk of complicated grieving
- Impaired mood regulation
- Powerlessness
- Risk of powerlessness
- Readiness for enhanced power
- Impaired resilience
- Risk for impaired resilience
- Readiness for enhanced resilience
- Chronic sorrow
- Stress overload
- Acute substance withdrawal syndrome
- Risk of acute substance withdrawal syndrome
- Decisional conflict
- Impaired emancipated decision-making
- Risk of impaired emancipated decision-making
- Readiness for enhanced emancipated decision-making
- Moral distress
- Impaired religiosity
- Risk of impaired religiosity
- Readiness for enhanced religiosity
- Spiritual distress
- Risk of spiritual distress
- Risk of other-directed violence
- Risk of self-directed violence

19

Contd...

- Parental role conflict
- Ineffective role performance
- Impaired social interaction
- Sexual dysfunction
- Ineffective sexuality pattern
- Risk of self-mutilation
- Risk of suicide

Objectives for Psychiatric Clinical Posting

Description of the Mental Hospital

1. Brief History of an Institution

....

....

....

....

....

....

....

....

....

2. Objectives of an Institution

....

....

....

....

....

....

....

....

3. Departments Available in the Institution

4. Functions of the Institution

Psychiatric OPD

Psychiatric History Collection-1

1. Identification Data

Name of the patient   : ....

Father/Husband name   : ....

Age   : .... Sex : ....

Ward admitted in   : ....

Diagnosis   : ....

Date of admission   : ....

Marital status   : ....

Religion   : ....

Nationality   : ....

Educational status   : ....

Occupation   : ....

Family income/month   : ....

Mode of admission   : ....Voluntary/Brought by relatives/Through court/Through police

2. Informant

Name of the informant   : ....

Relation with patient   : ....

Duration of stay with patient : .... :

3. Presenting Chief Complaints

....

....

....

....

....

....

....

....

4. History of Present Illness
(Duration, mode of onset, course of illness, intensity, precipitating factors, associated disturbances, etc.)

....

....

....

....

....

....

....

....

....

5. Past Psychiatric History
(Past psychiatric problems, hospitalization, treatment history, previous episode of presenting complaints)

....

....

....

....

....

....

....

....

6. Past Medical History
(Past medical problems, hospitalization, treatment history, surgery, if any, etc.)

....

....

....

....

....

....

....

....

....

7. Family History

Type of family: Nuclear/Joint

Brief description of family: (Parents, siblings, spouse, children)

Genogram

....

....

....

....

....

....

....

....

Family psychiatric history

(Behavioral/emotional problems in any family member, drugs/Alcohol abuse in family, etc.)

....

....

....

....

....

....

....

....

....

8. Personal History

a. **Perinatal history:**

    Antenatal period

       Pregnancy :   Eventful/Uneventful

    Intranatal

       Delivery   :   Normal/LSCS/Forceps

       Birth cry   :   Immediate/Delayed

       Complications : ....

    Postnatal

       Birth defects   : ....

       Complications   : ....

b. **Childhood history:**

    Relation of parents with child : ....

    Relationship with siblings   : ....

    Relationship with other children: ....

    Developmental milestones   : ....

Use of defense mechanisms : ....

Behavioral and emotional problems:...

c. Educational history:

Age of joining the school : ....

Academic performance : ....

Attitude toward teachers : ....

Relation with peers : ....

School attendance : ....

School phobia : ....

Conduct disorders : ....

d. Play history:

Types of games played : ....

Relation with playmates : ....

e. Emotional problems during adolescence:

Running away from home : ....Yes/No

Delinquency : ....Yes/No

Smoking : ....Yes/No

Alcohol/any other drug : ....Yes/No

f. Puberty:

Age of appearance of secondary sexual characteristics: ....

Anxiety related to puberty changes: ....

Age of menarche : ....

Regularity of cycle : ....

Menstrual problems (if any):..

g. Obstetrical history:

LMP : ....

Parity : ....

No. of living children: ....

Termination of pregnancy (if any): ....

h. Occupational history:

Age at starting work : ....

Jobs held in chronological order: ....

Reason for change in jobs: ....

Current job satisfaction : ....

Relation with workmates : ....

Appropriateness of job to patient: ....

i. Sexual and marital history:

Type of marriage : ....

Duration of marriage : ....

Interpersonal relation with spouse: ....

Sexual relation with spouse: ....

j. Premorbid personality:

Interpersonal relationship : ....

Family and social relationship: ....

Use of leisure time : ....

Predominant mood : ....

      Optimistic/Pessimistic

      Stable/Fluctuating

      Cheerful/Despondent

Reaction to life stressors : ....

Attitude toward self : ....

Attitude toward others : ....

Attitude toward work/responsibility: ....

Religious beliefs and rituals: ....

Fantasy life : ....

Habits : ....

Hobbies : ....

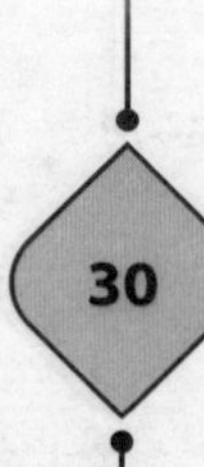

Psychiatric History Collection 2

1. Identification Data

Name of the patient : ....

Father/Husband name : ....

Age : .... Sex : ....

Ward admitted in : ....

Diagnosis : ....

Date of admission : ....

Marital status : ....

Religion : ....

Nationality : ....

Educational status : ....

Occupation : ....

Family income/month : ....

Mode of admission : ....Voluntary/Brought by relatives/Through court/Through police

2. Informant

Name of the informant : ....

Relation with patient : ....

Duration of stay with patient : .... :

3. Presenting Chief Complaints

....

....

....

....

4. History of Present Illness
(Duration, mode of onset, course of illness, intensity, precipitating factors, associated disturbances, etc.)

5. Past Psychiatric History
(Past psychiatric problems, hospitalization, treatment history, previous episode of presenting complaints)

....

....

6. Past Medical History
(Past medical problems, hospitalization, treatment history, surgery if any, etc.)

....

....

....

....

....

....

....

....

....

7. Family History

Type of family: Nuclear/Joint

Brief description of family: (Parents, siblings, spouse, children)

....

....

....

....

....

....

....

Genogram

....

....

Family psychiatric history

(Behavioral/emotional problems in any family member, drugs/alcohol abuse in family, etc.)

....

....

....

....

....

....

....

....

....

8. Personal History

a. **Perinatal history:**

    Antenatal period

      Pregnancy :   Eventful/Uneventful

    Intranatal

      Delivery   :   Normal/LSCS/Forceps

      Birth cry   :   Immediate/Delayed

      Complications : ....

    Postnatal

      Birth defects   : ....

      Complications : ....

b. **Childhood history:**

Relation of parents with child : ....

Relationship with siblings   : ....

Relationship with other children : ....

Developmental milestones : ....

Use of defense mechanisms   : ....

Behavioral and emotional problems: ....

c. Educational history:

Age of joining the school   : ....

Academic performance   : ....

Attitude toward teachers   : ....

Relation with peers   : ....

School attendance   : ....

School phobia   : ....

Conduct disorders   : ....

d. Play history:

Types of games played   : ....

Relation with playmates   : ....

e. Emotional problems during adolescence:

Running away from home   : ....Yes/No

Delinquency   : ....Yes/No

Smoking   : ....Yes/No

Alcohol/any other drug   : ....Yes/No

f. Puberty:

Age of appearance of secondary sexual characteristics: ....

Anxiety related to puberty changes: ....

Age of menarche   : ....

Regularity of cycle   : ....

Menstrual problems (if any): ....

g. Obstetrical history:

LMP   : ....

Parity   : ....

No. of living children: ....

Termination of pregnancy (if any): ....

h. Occupational history:

Age at starting work : ....

Jobs held in chronological order: ....

Reason for change in jobs: ....

Current job satisfaction : ....

Relation with workmates : ....

Appropriateness of job to patient: ....

i. Sexual and marital history:

Type of marriage : ....

Duration of marriage : ....

Interpersonal relation with spouse: ....

Sexual relation with spouse: ....

j. Premorbid personality:

Interpersonal relationship : ....

Family and social relationship: ....

Use of leisure time : ....

Predominant mood : ....

        Optimistic/Pessimistic

        Stable/Fluctuating

        Cheerful/Despondent

Reaction to life stressors : ....

Attitude toward self : ....

Attitude toward others : ....

Attitude toward work/responsibility: ....

Religious beliefs and rituals: ....

Fantasy life : ....

Habits : ....

Hobbies : ....

Mental Status Examination-1

1. Identification Data

Name of the patient   : ....

Father/Husband name : ....

Age   : .... Sex : ....

Ward admitted in   : ....

Date of admission   : ....

Marital status   : ....

Religion   : ....

Nationality   : ....

Educational status   : ....

Occupation   : ....

Family income/month : ....

Languages known   : ....

A. General appearance and behavior:

Appearance   : ....

Level of grooming   : ....

Level of cleanliness : ....

Level of consciousness: ....

Mode of entry   : ....

Cooperativeness   : ....

Eye to eye contact   : ....

Psychomotor activity : ....

Rapport   : ....

Gestures   : ....

Posture   : ....

Other movements   : ....

Catatonic phenomena : ....

B. Speech:

Initiation : ....

Reaction time : ....

Rate : ....

Productivity : ....

Volume : ....

Tone : ....

Relevance : ....

Stream : ....

Coherence : ....

Others : ....

Sample of speech : ....

....

....

....

....

....

....

....

C. Mood and affect:

Subjective mood : ....

Objective mood (affect) : ....

Appropriateness : ....

Intensity : ....

Type : ....

Range : ....

Stability : ....

D. Thought:

Stream of thought : ....

Form : ....

Content : ....

Delusions : ....

Ideas : ....

Thought alienation : ....

Obsessions : ....

Phobias (specify) : ....

E. Perception:

- Illusions : ....Present/Absent

- Hallucinations : ....Present/Absent

- If yes : ....Auditory/Visual/Olfactory/Gustatory/Tactile

- Somatic passivity : ....Present/Absent

- Depersonalization : ....Present/Absent

- Derealization : ....Present/Absent

F. Cognitive functions:

i. Consciousness : ....Conscious/Cloudy/Comatosed

ii. Orientation

- ◆ Time : Oriented/Disoriented
- ◆ Place : Oriented/Disoriented
- ◆ Person : Oriented/Disoriented

iii. Attention and concentration:

- ◆ Arousal : Normal/Difficulty
- ◆ Digit forward test : ....
  (7: Good average
  6: Low average
  5: Marginal)

- ◆ Digit backward test : ....
  (5: Average
  4: Marginal)

- ◆ Names of the months forward : ....
- ◆ Names of the months backward : ....

    ◆ **Attention** : Intact/Altered

    ◆ **Concentration** : Intact/Altered

iv. **Memory**

    ◆ **Immediate** : ....Intact/Altered

(Repetition of three non-related

words and recall after three minutes.)

    ◆ **Recent** : ....Intact/Altered

(Occurences in past 24 hours) ....

    ◆ **Remote** : ....Intact/Altered

(Personal events, illness related events)

v. **Intelligence**

    ◆ General information : ....Intact/Altered

    ◆ Arithmetic ability : ....Intact/Altered

vi. **Abstraction**

    ◆ Interpretation of proverbs : ....

    ◆ Similarities between paired objects : ....

    ◆ Dissimilarities between paired objects: ....

    ◆ **Abstraction** : Intact/Altered

vii. **Judgment**

    ◆ Personal : Intact/Impaired

    ◆ Social : Intact/Impaired

    ◆ Test : Intact/Impaired

G. Insight

    ▪ Awareness of abnormal behavior: Yes/No/Maybe

    ▪ Attribution to physical cause : Yes/No/Maybe

    ▪ Willingness to take treatment : Yes/No/Maybe

H. Diagnostic formulation : ....

....

....

....

....

....

....

Mental Status Examination-2

1. Identification Data

Name of the patient : ....

Father/Husband name : ....

Age : .... Sex : ....

Ward admitted in : ....

Date of admission : ....

Marital status : ....

Religion : ....

Nationality : ....

Educational status : ....

Occupation : ....

Family income/month : ....

Languages known : ....

A. General appearance and behavior:

Appearance : ....

Level of grooming : ....

Level of cleanliness : ....

Level of consciousness: ....

Mode of entry : ....

Cooperativeness : ....

Eye to eye contact : ....

Psychomotor activity : ....

Rapport : ....

Gestures : ....

Posture : ....

Other movements : ....

Catatonic phenomena: ....

B. Speech:

Initiation : ....

Reaction time : ....

Rate : ....

Productivity : ....

Volume : ....

Tone : ....

Relevance : ....

Stream : ....

Coherence : ....

Others : ....

Sample of speech : ....

....

....

....

....

....

....

....

....

C. Mood and affect:

Subjective mood : ....

Objective mood (affect) : ....

Appropriateness : ....

Intensity : ....

Type : ....

Range : ....

Stability : ....

D. Thought:

Stream of thought : ....

Form : ....

Content : ....

Delusions : ....

Ideas : ....

Thought alienation : ....

Obsessions : ....

Phobias (specify) : ....

E. Perception:

- Illusions : ....Present/Absent
- Hallucinations : ....Present/Absent
- If yes : ....Auditory/Visual/Olfactory/Gustatory/Tactile
- Somatic passivity : ....Present/Absent
- Depersonalization : ....Present/Absent
- Derealization : ....Present/Absent

F. Cognitive functions:

i. Consciousness : ....Conscious/Cloudy/Comatosed

ii. Orientation

- Time : Oriented/Disoriented
- Place : Oriented/Disoriented
- Person : Oriented/Disoriented

iii. Attention and concentration:

- Arousal : Normal/Difficulty
- Digit forward test : ....
  (7: Good average
  6: Low average
  5: Marginal)
- Digit backward test : ....
  (5: Average
  4: Marginal)
- Names of the months forward : ....
- Names of the months backward : ....
- **Attention** : Intact/Altered
- **Concentration** : Intact/Altered

    iv. Memory

- **Immediate** : ....Intact/Altered
(Repetition of three non-related
words and recall after three minutes.)
- **Recent** : ....Intact/Altered
(Occurences in past 24 hours) ....
- **Remote** : ....Intact/Altered
(Personal events, illness related events)

    v. Intelligence

- General information : ....Intact/Altered
- Arithmetic ability : ....Intact/Altered

   vi. Abstraction

- Interpretation of proverbs : ....
- Similarities between paired objects : ....
- Dissimilarities between paired objects: ....
- **Abstraction** : Intact/Altered

  vii. Judgment

- Personal : Intact/Impaired
- Social : Intact/Impaired
- Test : Intact/Impaired

G. Insight

- Awareness of abnormal behavior: Yes/No/Maybe
- Attribution to physical cause : Yes/No/Maybe
- Willingness to take treatment : Yes/No/Maybe

H. Diagnostic formulation : ....

....

....

....

....

....

....

Mini Mental Status Examination-1

1. Identification Data

Name of the patient   : ....

Father/Husband name : ....

Age   : .... Sex : ....

Ward admitted in   : ....

Diagnosis   : ....

Date of admission   : ....

Marital status   : ....

Religion   : ....

Nationality   : ....

Educational status   : ....

Occupation   : ....

Family income/month   : ....

Languages known   : ....

Sl. no.		Components	Time	Score	Patient's score
		Orientation			
1.	a.	What year is this?	10 seconds	1	
	b.	Which season is this?	10 seconds	1	
	c.	What month is this?	10 seconds	1	
	d.	What is today's date?	10 seconds	1	
	e.	What day of the week is this?	10 seconds	1	
2.	a.	What country are we in?	10 seconds	1	
	b.	What district are we in?	10 seconds	1	
	c.	What city/town are we in?	10 seconds	1	
	d.	In home: What is the address of this house? In hospital: What is the name of this building?	10 seconds	1	
	e.	In home: What room are we in? In hospital: What floor are we on?	10 seconds	1	

Contd...

Sl. no.		Components	Time	Score	Patient's score
3.		Say name of the three objects to a patient. Ask him/her to repeat when you finished 3 object names And also ask him/her to remember what are they and ask him/her to name them again in a few minutes. Say the following words slowly at 1 second intervals—umbrella/car/woman	20 seconds	3	
		Attention			
4.		Spell the word India and ask him/her to spell it backward. or Subtract serials of 7 from 100 (5 subtractions)	30 seconds	5	
		Recall			
5.		Now ask what were the three objects which you have asked him to remember?	10 seconds	3	
		Language			
6.		Show cell phone. Ask: What is this called?	10 seconds	1	
7.		Show pencil. Ask: What is this called?	10 seconds	1	
8.		Say any phrase and ask him/her to repeat the phrase after you.	10 seconds	1	
9.		Say: Read the words written on the page and then do what it says. Then handover the person the sheet/paper with "close your eyes" written over it. If the person reads and does not close his eyes after reading, repeat up to three times. Score only if subject closes eyes.	10 seconds	1	
10.		Ask the person to write any complete sentence on that piece of paper. (**Note:** The sentence must make sense. Ignore spelling errors.)	30 seconds	1	
11.		Place design, eraser and pencil in front of the person. **Say:** Copy this design please. Allow multiple tries. Wait until person is finished and hands it back. Score only for correctly copied diagram with a 4-sided figure between two 5-sided figures.	1 minute	1	
12.		**Ask** the person if he/she is right or left-handed. Take a piece of paper and hold it up in front of the person. **Say:** Take this paper in your right/left hand (whichever is non-dominant), fold the paper in half once with both hands and put the paper down on the floor. Score 1 point for each instruction executed correctly.	30 seconds	1	
		Takes paper correctly in hand.		1	

Contd...

Sl. no.		Components	Time	Score	Patient's score
		Folds it in half.		1	
		Puts it on the floor.		1	
		Total test score		30	

Inference

Interpretation

Method	Score	Interpretation
Severity	24–30	No cognitive impairment
	18–23	Mild cognitive impairment
	0–17	Severe cognitive impairment

Mini Mental Status Examination-2

1. Identification Data

Name of the patient : ....

Father/Husband name : ....

Age : .... Sex : ....

Ward admitted in : ....

Diagnosis : ....

Date of admission : ....

Marital status : ....

Religion : ....

Nationality : ....

Educational status : ....

Occupation : ....

Family income/month : ....

Languages known : ....

Sl. no.		Components	Time	Score	Patient's score
		Orientation			
1.	a.	What year is this?	10 seconds	1	
	b.	Which season is this?	10 seconds	1	
	c.	What month is this?	10 seconds	1	
	d.	What is today's date?	10 seconds	1	
	e.	What day of the week is this?	10 seconds	1	
2.	a.	What country are we in?	10 seconds	1	
	b.	What district are we in?	10 seconds	1	
	c.	What city/town are we in?	10 seconds	1	
	d.	In home: What is the address of this house? In hospital: What is the name of this building?	10 seconds	1	
	e.	In home: What room are we in? In hospital: What floor are we on?	10 seconds	1	

Contd...

Sl. no.		Components	Time	Score	Patient's score
3.		Say name of the three objects to a patient. Ask him/her to repeat when you finished 3 object names And also ask him/her to remember what are they and ask him/her to name them again in a few minutes. Say the following words slowly at 1 second intervals— umbrella/car/woman	20 seconds	3	
		Attention			
4.		Spell the word India and ask him/her to spell it backward. or Subtract serials of 7 from 100 (5 subtractions)	30 seconds	5	
		Recall			
5.		Now ask what were the three objects which you have asked him to remember?	10 seconds	3	
		Language			
6.		Show cell phone. Ask: What is this called?	10 seconds	1	
7.		Show pencil. Ask: What is this called?	10 seconds	1	
8.		Say any phrase and ask him/her to repeat the phrase after you.	10 seconds	1	
9.		Say: Read the words written on the page and then do what it says. Then handover the person the sheet/paper with "close your eyes" written over it. If the person reads and does not close his eyes after reading, repeat up to three times. Score only if subject closes eyes.	10 seconds	1	
10.		Ask the person to write any complete sentence on that piece of paper. (**Note:** The sentence must make sense. Ignore spelling errors.)	30 seconds	1	
11.		Place design, eraser and pencil in front of the person. **Say:** Copy this design please. Allow multiple tries. Wait until person is finished and hands it back. Score only for correctly copied diagram with a 4-sided figure between two 5-sided figures.	1 minute	1	
12.		**Ask** the person if he/she is right or left-handed. Take a piece of paper and hold it up in front of the person. **Say:** Take this paper in your right/left hand (whichever is non-dominant), fold the paper in half once with both hands and put the paper down on the floor. Score 1 point for each instruction executed correctly.	30 seconds	1	
		Takes paper correctly in hand.		1	

Contd...

Sl. no.		Components	Time	Score	Patient's score
		Folds it in half.		1	
		Puts it on the floor.		1	
		Total test score		30	
		Puts it on the floor.		1	
		Total test score		30	

Inference

Interpretation

Method	Score	Interpretation
Severity	24–30	No cognitive impairment
	18–23	Mild cognitive impairment
	0–17	Severe cognitive impairment

Health Education-1

Topic   : ....

Group   : ....

Size of the group   : ....

Method of teaching   : ....

Medium of teaching   : ....

Audio-visual aids   : ....

Duration   : ....

Venue   : ....

1. General objectives

....

....

....

....

....

....

....

....

....

2. Specific objectives

....

....

....

Time	Specific Objectives	Contents	Activities		A-V aids	Method of evaluation
			Teacher	Clients		

Contd...

Time	Specific Objectives	Contents	Activities		A-V aids	Method of evaluation
			Teacher	Clients		

Observation Report of Visit to Psychiatric OPD

1. Introduction of the institution

....

....

....

....

....

....

....

2. Brief description of OPD

....

....

....

....

....

....

....

3. General objectives of the OPD

....

....

....

....

....

Time	Specific Objectives	Contents	Activities		A-V aids	Method of evaluation
			Teacher	Clients		

....

....

4. Different OPDs available

1.		9.	
2.		10.	
3.		11.	
4.		12.	
5.		13.	
6.		14.	
7.		15.	
8.		16.	

5. Staffing pattern of OPD

....

....

....

....

....

....

....

6. General functions of OPD

....

....

....

....

....

....

....

7. Summary of the visit

....

....

....

....

....

....

....

Child Guidance Clinic

Observation Report of Visit to Child Guidance Clinic

1. Introduction of child guidance clinic

2. General objectives

3. Functions of child guidance clinic

....

....

4. Staffing pattern of child guidance clinic

....

....

....

....

....

....

....

5. Summary of the visit

....

....

....

....

....

....

....

....

History Collection and Mental Status Examination-1

1. Identification Data

Name of the patient : ....

Father/Husband name : ....

Age : ....Sex : ....

Ward admitted in : ....

Diagnosis : ....

Date of admission : ....

Marital status : ....

Religion : ....

Nationality : ....

Educational status : ....

Occupation : ....

Family income/month : ....

Mode of admission : ....Voluntary/Brought by relatives/Through court/Through police

2. Informant

Name of the informant :..

Relation with patient :..

Duration of stay with patient :..

3. Presenting Chief Complaints

....

....

....

....

4. History of Present Illness
(Duration, mode of onset, course of illness, intensity, precipitating factors, associated disturbances, etc.)

5. Past Psychiatric History
(Past psychiatric problems, hospitalization, treatment history, previous episode of presenting complaints)

6. Past Medical History
(Past medical problems, hospitalization, treatment history, surgery, if any, etc.)

....

....

....

....

....

....

....

7. Family History

Genogram

Type of family: Nuclear/Joint
Brief description of family: (Parents, siblings, spouse, children)

....

....

....

....

....

....

Family psychiatric history
(Behavioral/Emotional problems in any family member, drugs/Alcohol abuse in family, etc.)

....

....

....

....

....

....

....

8. Personal History

a. Perinatal history:

Antenatal period

Pregnancy	:	Eventful/Uneventful

Intranatal

Delivery	:	Normal/LSCS/Forceps
Birth cry	:	Immediate/Delayed
Complications	:	....

Postnatal

Birth defects	:	....
Complications	:	....

b. Childhood history:

Relation of parents with child : ....

Relationship with siblings : ....

Relationship with other children : ....

Developmental milestones : ....

Use of defense mechanisms : ....

Behavioral and emotional problems : ....

c. Educational history:

Age of joining the school : ....

Academic performance : ....

Attitude toward teachers : ....

Relation with peers : ....

School attendance : ....

School phobia : ....

Conduct disorders : ....

d. Play history:

Types of games played : ....

Relation with playmates : ....

e. Emotional problems during adolescence:

Running away from home : ....Yes/No

Delinquency : ....Yes/No

Smoking : ....Yes/No

Alcohol/any other drug : ....Yes/No

f. Puberty:

Age of appearance of secondary sexual characteristics: ....

Anxiety related to puberty changes: ....

Age of menarche : ....

Regularity of cycle : ....

Menstrual problems (if any): ....

g. Premorbid personality:

Interpersonal relationship : ....

Family and social relationship : ....

Use of leisure time : ....

Predominant mood : ....

Reaction to life stressors : ....

Attitude toward self : ....

Attitude toward others : ....

Attitude toward work/Responsibility: ....:

Religious beliefs and rituals : ....

Fantasy life : ....

Habits : ....

Hobbies : ....

Mental Status Examination

A. General appearance and behavior:

Appearance : ....

Level of grooming : ....

Level of cleanliness : ....

Level of consciousness	:	....
Mode of entry	:	....
Cooperativeness	:	....
Eye to eye contact	:	....
Psychomotor activity	:	....
Rapport	:	....
Gestures	:	....
Posture	:	....
Other movements	:	....
Catatonic phenomena	:	....

B. Speech:

....

....

....

....

....

....

....

C. Mood and affect:

....

....

....

....

....

....

D. Thought:

....

....

....

....

....

....

....

E. Perception:

....

....

....

....

....

....

....

F. Cognitive functions:

   i. Consciousness : ....

   ii. Orientation

      ◆ Time   : ....Oriented/Disoriented

      ◆ Place   : ....Oriented/Disoriented

      ◆ Person   : ....Oriented/Disoriented

   iii. Attention and concentration:

....

....

....

....

iv. Memory

v. Intelligence

vi. Abstraction

....

....

....

vii. Judgment

....

....

....

....

....

....

....

G. Insight

- Awareness of abnormal behavior : .... Yes/No/Maybe
- Attribution to physical cause : .... Yes/No/Maybe
- Willingness to take treatment : .... Yes/No/Maybe

H. Diagnostic formulation : ....

....

....

....

....

....

Observing and Assisting in Therapy-1

1. Identification Data

Name of the patient   : ....

Father/Husband name   : ....

Age   : .... Sex: ....

Ward admitted in   : ....

Diagnosis   : ....

2. History of present illness

....

....

....

....

....

....

....

....

3. Treatment

....

....

....

....

....

....

....

....

4. Details of psychotherapy

a. **Type of therapy indicated:**..

b. **Brief description of the therapy**

....

....

....

....

....

....

c. **Therapeutic approaches used**

....

....

....

....

....

d. **Uses of the therapy**

....

....

e. **Role of a nurse in the therapy**

5. Summary

Parental Health Education on Mental Deficiency

Topic   : ....

Group   : ....

Size of the group   : ....

Method of teaching : ....

Medium of teaching : ....

Audio-visual aids   : ....

Duration   : ....

1. General objectives

2. Specific objectives

Time	Specific Objectives	Contents	Activities		A-V aids	Method of evaluation
			Teacher	Clients		

Contd

Time	Specific Objectives	Contents	Activities		A-V aids	Method of evaluation
			Teacher	Clients		

Contd...

Time	Specific Objectives	Contents	Activities		A-V aids	Method of evaluation
			Teacher	Clients		

In-Patient Ward

Psychiatric History Collection and Mental Status examination

1. Identification Data

Name of the patient : ....

Father/Husband name : ....

Age : .... Sex : ....

Ward admitted in : ....

Diagnosis : ....

Date of admission : ....

Marital status : ....

Religion : ....

Nationality : ....

Educational status : ....

Occupation : ....

Family income/month : ....

Mode of admission : .... Voluntary/Brought by relatives/Through court/Through police

2. Informant

Name of the informant : ....

Relation with patient : ....

Duration of stay with patient : ....

3. Presenting Chief Complaints

....

....

....

....

....

....

....

....

4. History of Present Illness
(Duration, mode of onset, course of illness, intensity, precipitating factors, associated disturbances, etc.)

....

....

....

....

....

....

....

5. Past Psychiatric History
(Past psychiatric problems, hospitalization, treatment history, previous episode of presenting complaints)

....

....

....

....

....

....

....

6. Past Medical History
(Past medical problems, hospitalization, treatment history, surgery, if any, etc.)

....

....

....

....

....

....

....

....

7. Family History

Genogram

Type of family: Nuclear/Joint
Brief description of family: (Parents, siblings, spouse, children)

....

....

....

....

....

....

....

Family psychiatric history
(Behavioral/Emotional problems in any family member, drugs/Alcohol abuse in family, etc.)

....

....

....

....

....

....

....

....

....

....

....

8. Personal History

a. **Antenatal period**

Pregnancy	:	Eventful/Uneventful

Intranatal

Delivery	:	Normal/LSCS/Forceps
Birth cry	:	Immediate/Delayed
Complications	:	....

Postnatal

Birth defects	:	....
Complications	:	....

b. **Childhood history:**

Relation of parents with child : ....

Relationship with siblings : ....

Relationship with other children : ....

Developmental milestones : ....

Use of defense mechanisms : ....

Behavioral and emotional problems : ....

c. **Educational history:**

Age of joining the school : ....

Academic performance : ....

Attitude toward teachers : ....

Relation with peers : ....

School attendance : ....

School phobia : ....

Conduct disorders : ....

d. Play history:

Types of games played : ....

Relation with playmates : ....

e. Emotional problems during adolescence:

Running away from home : ....Yes/No

Delinquency : ....Yes/No

Smoking : ....Yes/No

Alcohol/any other drug : ....Yes/No

f. Puberty:

Age of appearance of secondary sexual characteristics: ....

Anxiety related to puberty changes : ....

Age of menarche : ....

Regularity of cycle : ....

Menstrual problems (if any) : ....

g. Obstetrical history:

LMP : ....

Parity : ....

No. of living children : ....

Termination of pregnancy (if any) : ....

h. Occupational history:

Age at starting work : ....

Jobs held in chronological order : ....

Reason for change in jobs : ....

Current job satisfaction : ....

Relation with workmates : ....

Appropriateness of job to patient : ....

i. Sexual and marital history:

Type of marriage : ....

Duration of marriage : ....

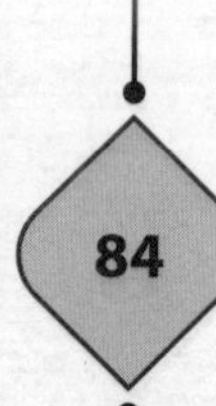

Interpersonal relation with spouse : ....

Sexual relation with spouse   : ....

j. Premorbid personality:

Interpersonal relationship   : ....

Family and social relationship   : ....

Use of leisure time   : ....

Predominant mood   Optimistic/Pessimistic

                               Stable/Fluctuating

                               Cheerful/Despondent

Reaction to life stressors   : ....

Attitude toward self   : ....

Attitude toward others   : ....

Attitude toward work/responsibility : ....

Religious beliefs and rituals   : ....

Fantasy life   : ....

Habits   : ....

Hobbies   : ....

Mental Status Examination

A. General appearance and behavior:

Appearance   : ....

Level of grooming   : ....

Level of cleanliness   : ....

Level of consciousness : ....

Mode of entry   : ....

Cooperativeness   : ....

Eye to eye contact   : ....

Psychomotor activity   : ....

Rapport   : ....

Gestures   : ....

Posture   : ....

Other movements   : ....

Catatonic phenomena : ....

B. Speech:

....

....

....

....

....

....

....

C. Mood and affect:

....

....

....

....

....

....

D. Thought:

....

....

....

....

....

....

....

E. Perception:

....

....

....

....

....

....

F. Cognitive functions:

   i. Consciousness : ....

   ii. Orientation

      ◆ Time : ....Oriented/Disoriented

      ◆ Place : ....Oriented/Disoriented

      ◆ Person : ....Oriented/Disoriented

   iii. Attention and concentration

....

....

....

....

....

....

....

   iv. Memory

....

....

v. Intelligence

vi. Abstraction

vii. Judgment

....
....
....
....
....
....

G. Insight:

- Awareness of abnormal behavior : .... Yes/No/Maybe
- Attribution to physical cause : .... Yes/No/Maybe
- Willingness to take treatment : .... Yes/No/Maybe

H. Diagnostic formulation : ....

....
....
....
....
....
....

Psychiatric Care Study

1. Identification Data

Name of the patient : ....

Father/Husband name : ....

Age : .... Sex:

Ward admitted in : ....

Diagnosis : ....

Date of admission : ....

Marital status : ....

Religion : ....

Nationality : ....

Educational status : ....

Occupation : ....

Family income/month : ....

Mode of admission : .... Voluntary/Brought by relatives/Through court/Through police

2. Informant

Name of the informant : ....

Relation with patient : ....

Duration of stay with patient : ....

3. Presenting Chief Complaints

....

....

....

....

....

....

....

....

4. History of Present Illness
(Duration, mode of onset, course of illness, intensity, precipitating factors, associated disturbances, etc.)

....

....

....

....

....

....

....

....

5. Past Psychiatric History
(Past psychiatric problems, hospitalization, treatment history, previous episode of presenting complaints)

....

....

....

....

....

....

....

6. Past Medical History
(Past medical problems, hospitalization, treatment history, surgery, if any, etc.)

....

....

....

....

....

7. Family History

Genogram

Type of family: Nuclear/Joint
Brief Description of family: (Parents, siblings, spouse, children)

....

....

....

....

....

....

....

....

Family psychiatric history
(Behavioral/Emotional problems in any family member, drugs/Alcohol abuse in family, etc.)

....

....

....

....

....

8. Personal History (Only significant in brief)

....

....

....

....

....

....

9. Mental Status Examination (Significant findings in brief)

A. General appearance and behavior

....

....

....

....

....

B. Speech

....

....

....

....

....

....

C. Mood and affect

    Subjective mood   : ....

    Objective mood (affect)   : ....

....

....

....

....

....

D. Thought

....

....

....

....

....

....

E. Perception

....

....

....

....

....

....

....

....

F. Cognitive functions

i. Consciousness : .... Conscious/Cloudy/Comatose

ii. Orientation

- Time : ....Oriented/Disoriented
- Place : ....Oriented/Disoriented
- Person : ....Oriented/Disoriented

iii. Attention and concentration

- Arousal : .... Normal/Difficulty
- Attention : ....Intact/Altered
- Concentration : ....Intact/Altered

iv. Memory

- Immediate : ....Intact/Altered
- Recent : ....Intact/Altered
- Remote : ....Intact/Altered

v. Intelligence

- General information : ....Intact/Altered
- Arithmetic ability : ....Intact/Altered

vi. Abstraction

- Interpretation of proverbs : ....
- Similarities between paired objects : ....
- Dissimilarities between paired objects: ....
- Abstraction : Intact/Altered

vii. Judgment

- Personal : .... Intact/Impaired
- Social : .... Intact/Impaired
- Test : .... Intact/Impaired

G. Insight

- Awareness of abnormal behavior: ....Yes/No/Maybe
- Attribution to physical cause : ....Yes/No/Maybe
- Willingness to take treatment : ....Yes/No/Maybe

10. Physical Examination (Significant findings)

A. Anthropometric measurements

- Height : ....
- Weight : ....
- Head circumference : ....
- Chest circumference : ....
- Mid-arm circumference : ....

B. General appearance

....

....

....

....

....

....

C. Head-to-toe examination (significant findings, if any)

....

....

....

....

....

....

....

....

....

11. Investigations

Sl. no.	Investigation	Normal value	Patient's value	Inference

12. Medical Treatment

Sl. no.	Drug	Action	Dose	Frequency	Route

Contd...

Sl. no.	Drug	Action	Dose	Frequency	Route

13. ECT (If any)

....

....

....

....

....

....

....

14. Psychological Therapy (If any)

....
....
....
....
....
....
....
....

15. Comparison Between Patient and Book Picture

Definition of disease

Contd...

Patient picture	Book picture
Clinical features	
Psychopathology	
Diagnostic evaluation	
Management	
Prognosis	

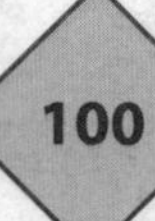

16. List of Nursing Diagnosis

....

....

....

....

....

....

....

....

....

....

17. Nursing Care Plan

Nursing diagnosis:
Goal/Expected outcome

Contd...

Assessment	Intervention	Implementation	Evaluation

Nursing diagnosis:

Goal/Expected outcome

Assessment	Intervention	Implementation	Evaluation

Nursing diagnosis:

Goal/Expected outcome

Assessment	Intervention	Implementation	Evaluation

Nursing diagnosis:

Goal/Expected outcome

Assessment	Intervention	Implementation	Evaluation

18. Health Education

19. Conclusion

Psychiatric Case Presentation

1. Identification Data

Name of the patient :...

Father/Husband name :...

Age :...Sex: ....

Ward admitted in :...

Diagnosis :...

Date of admission :...

Marital status :...

Religion :...

Nationality :...

Educational status :...

Occupation :...

Family income/month :...

Mode of admission :...Voluntary/Brought by relatives/through court/through police

2. Informant

Name of the informant :...

Relation with patient :...

Duration of stay with patient :...

3. Presenting Chief Complaints

....

....

....

....

....

....

....

....

4. History of Present Illness
(Duration, mode of onset, course of illness, intensity, precipitating factors, associated disturbances, etc.)

....

....

....

....

....

....

....

5. Past Psychiatric History
(Past psychiatric problems, hospitalization, treatment history, previous episode of presenting complaints)

....

....

....

....

....

....

6. Past Medical History

(Past medical problems, hospitalization, treatment history, surgery if any, etc.)

....

....

....

....

....

7. Family History

Type of family: Nuclear/Joint

Brief description of family: (Parents, siblings, spouse, children)

....

....

....

....

....

....

....

....

Genogram

Family psychiatric history

(Behavioral/emotional problems in any family member, drugs/alcohol abuse in family, etc.)

....

....

....

....

....

....

8. Personal History (Only significant in brief)

....

....

....

....

....

....

....

9. Mental Status Examination (Significant findings in brief)

A. General appearance and behavior

....

....

....

....

....

....

....

B. Speech

....

....

....

....

....

....

....

C. Mood and affect

Subjective mood   : ....

Objective mood (affect) : ....

....

....

....

....

....

D. Thought

....

....

....

....

....

....

E. Perception

....

....

....

....

....

....

....

F. Cognitive functions

  i. Consciousness   :.. Conscious/Cloudy/Comatose

  ii. Orientation

     ♦ Time   :...Oriented/Disoriented

     ♦ Place   :...Oriented/Disoriented

     ♦ Person   :...Oriented/Disoriented

  iii. Attention and concentration

     ♦ Arousal   :... Normal/Difficulty

     ♦ Attention   :...Intact/Altered

     ♦ Concentration   :...Intact/Altered

  iv. Memory

     ♦ Immediate   :...Intact/Altered

     ♦ Recent   :...Intact/Altered

     ♦ Remote   :...Intact/Altered

  v. Intelligence

     ♦ General information   :...Intact/Altered

     ♦ Arithmetic ability   :...Intact/Altered

  vi. Abstraction

     ♦ Interpretation of proverbs   :...

     ♦ Similarities between paired objects :...

     ♦ Dissimilarities between paired objects:...

     ♦ Abstraction : Intact/Altered

  vii. Judgment

     ♦ Personal   :... Intact/Impaired

     ♦ Social   :... Intact/Impaired

     ♦ Test   :... Intact/Impaired

G. Insight

  • Awareness of abnormal behavior:...Yes/No/Maybe

  • Attribution to physical cause   :...Yes/No/Maybe

  • Willingness to take treatment   :...Yes/No/Maybe

10. Physical Examination (Significant findings)

A. Anthropometric measurements

- Height : ....
- Weight : ....
- Head circumference : ....
- Chest circumference : ....
- Mid-arm circumference : ....

B. General appearance

....
....
....
....
....
....
....

C. Head-to-toe examination (significant findings if any)

....
....
....
....
....
....
....
....
....
....

11. Investigations

Sl. no.	Investigation	Normal value	Patient's value	Inference

12. Medical Treatment

Sl. no.	Drug	Action	Dose	Frequency	Route

Contd...

Sl. no.	Drug	Action	Dose	Frequency	Route

13. ECT (If any)

....

....

....

....

....

....

....

....

14. Psychological Therapy (If any)

....

....

....

....

....

....

....

....

15. Comparison Between Patient and Book Picture

Definition of disease

Contd...

Patient picture	Book picture
Clinical features	
Psychopathology	
Diagnostic evaluation	
Management	
Prognosis	

16. List of Nursing Diagnosis

....

....

....

....

....

....

....

....

....

....

17. Nursing Care Plan

Nursing diagnosis:

Goal/Expected outcome

Contd...

Assessment	Intervention	Implementation	Evaluation

Nursing diagnosis:

Goal/Expected outcome

Assessment	Intervention	Implementation	Evaluation

Nursing diagnosis:

Goal/Expected outcome

Assessment	Intervention	Implementation	Evaluation

Nursing diagnosis:

Goal/Expected outcome

Assessment	Intervention	Implementation	Evaluation

18. Health Education

19. Conclusion

Psychiatric Care Plan-1

1. Identification Data

Name of the patient   :..

Father/Husband name   :..

Age   :...Sex:.............................

Ward admitted in   :..

Diagnosis   :..

Date of admission   :..

Marital status   :..

Religion   :..

Nationality   :..

Educational status   :..

Occupation   :..

Family income/month   :..

Mode of admission   :...Voluntary/Brought by relatives/Through court/Through police

2. Informant

....

....

....

....

....

....

....

3. Presenting Chief Complaints

....

....

....

....

....

....

....

4. History of Present Illness
(Duration, mode of onset, course of illness, intensity, precipitating factors, associated disturbances, etc.)

....

....

....

....

....

....

....

5. Past Psychiatric History
(Past psychiatric problems, hospitalization, treatment history, previous episode of presenting complaints)

....

....

....

....

....

....

....

....

6. Past Medical History
(Past medical problems, hospitalization, treatment history, surgery if any, etc.)

....

....

....

....

....

....

....

7. Family History

....

....

....

....

....

....

Family psychiatric history

(Behavioral/emotional problems in any family member, drugs/alcohol abuse in family, etc.)

....

....

....

....

....

....

....

8. Personal History (Only significant in brief)

....

....

....

....

....

....

....

9. Mental Status Examination (Significant findings in brief)

A. General appearance and behavior

....

....

....

....

B. Speech

C. Mood and affect

D. Thought

....

....

....

....

E. Perception

....

....

....

....

....

....

....

F. Cognitive functions (consciousness, orientation, memory, attention, concentration, intelligence and abstract thinking)

....

....

....

....

....

....

G. Insight and Judgment

....

....

....

....

....

....

....

10. Physical examination (Significant findings)

A. Anthropometric measurements

- Height   : ....
- Weight   : ....
- Head circumference   : ....
- Chest circumference   : ....
- Mid-arm circumference : ....

B. General appearance

....

....

....

....

....

....

....

C. Head-to-toe examination (significant findings, if any)

....

....

....

....

....

....

....

11. Investigations

Sl. no.	Investigation	Normal value	Patient's value	Inference

12. Medical Treatment

Sl. no.	Drug	Action	Dose	Frequency	Route

Contd...

Sl. no.	Drug	Action	Dose	Frequency	Route

13. ECT/ Psychotherapies (if any)

....

....

....

....

....

....

....

14. List of Nursing Diagnosis

....

....

....

....

....

....

....

15. Nursing Care Plan

Nursing diagnosis:			
Goal/Expected outcome			
Assessment	Intervention	Implementation	Evaluation

Nursing diagnosis:

Goal/Expected outcome

Assessment	Intervention	Implementation	Evaluation

Nursing diagnosis:

Goal/Expected outcome

Assessment	Intervention	Implementation	Evaluation

Nursing diagnosis:

Goal/Expected outcome

Assessment	Intervention	Implementation	Evaluation

16. Health Education

Psychiatric Care Plan-2

1. Identification Data

Name of the patient   :..

Father/Husband name   :..

Age   :...Sex:..

Ward admitted in   :..

Diagnosis   :..

Date of admission   :..

Marital status   :..

Religion   :..

Nationality   :..

Educational status   :..

Occupation   :..

Family income/month   :..

Mode of admission   :...Voluntary/Brought by relatives/Through court/Through police

2. Informant

....

....

....

....

....

....

....

3. Presenting Chief Complaints

....

....

....

....

....

....

....

....

4. History of Present Illness
(Duration, mode of onset, course of illness, intensity, precipitating factors, associated disturbances, etc.)

....

....

....

....

....

....

....

5. Past Psychiatric History
(Past psychiatric problems, hospitalization, treatment history, previous episode of presenting complaints)

....

....

....

6. Past Medical History
(Past medical problems, hospitalization, treatment history, surgery if any, etc.)

7. Family History

Family psychiatric history

(Behavioral/emotional problems in any family member, drugs/alcohol abuse in family, etc.)

....

....

....

....

....

....

....

....

8. Personal History (Only significant in brief)

....

....

....

....

....

....

....

....

9. Mental Status Examination (Significant findings in brief)

A. General appearance and behavior

....

....

....

....

....

....

....

....

B. Speech

....

....

....

....

....

....

C. Mood and affect

....

....

....

....

....

D. Thought

....

....

....

E. Perception

F. Cognitive functions (consciousness, orientation, memory, attention, concentration, intelligence and abstract thinking)

G. Insight and Judgment

....

....

....

....

....

10. Physical examination (Significant findings)

A. Anthropometric measurements

- Height : ....
- Weight : ....
- Head circumference : ....
- Chest circumference : ....
- Mid-arm circumference : ....

B. General appearance

....

....

....

....

....

....

....

C. Head-to-toe examination (Significant findings if any)

....

....

....

....

....

....

....

11. Investigations

Sl. no.	Investigation	Normal value	Patient's value	Inference

12. Medical Treatment

Sl. no.	Drug	Action	Dose	Frequency	Route

13. ECT/ Psychotherapies (if any)

....

....

....

....

....

....

....

14. List of Nursing Diagnosis

....

....

....

....

....

....

....

....

15. Nursing Care Plan

Nursing diagnosis:

Goal/Expected outcome

Contd...

Assessment	Intervention	Implementation	Evaluation

Nursing diagnosis:

Goal/Expected outcome

Assessment	Intervention	Implementation	Evaluation

Nursing diagnosis:

Goal/Expected outcome

Assessment	Intervention	Implementation	Evaluation

Nursing diagnosis:

Goal/Expected outcome

Assessment	Intervention	Implementation	Evaluation

16. Health Education

Process Recording/Verbatim-1

1. Identification Data

Name of the patient   : ....

Father/Husband name   : ....

Age   : .... Sex: ....

Ward admitted in   : ....

Diagnosis   : ....

Date of admission   : ....

Marital status   : ....

Religion   : ....

Nationality   : ....

Educational status   : ....

Occupation   : ....

Family income/month   : ....

Languages known   : ....

2. Date of Verbatim   : ....

3. Place of verbatim   : ....

4. Situation   : ....

5. Objectives   : ....

....

....

....

....

....

....

....

Person	Verbal response	Nonverbal response	Inference

Contd...

Person	Verbal response	Nonverbal response	Inference

Summary

....

....

....

....

....

....

....

Time and place of next interview: ....

Process Recording/Verbatim-2

1. Identification Data

Name of the patient : ....

Father/husband name : ....

Age : .... Sex: ....

Ward admitted in : ....

Diagnosis : ....

Date of admission : ....

Marital status : ....

Religion : ....

Nationality : ....

Educational status : ....

Occupation : ....

Family income/month : ....

Languages known : ....

2. Date of Verbatim : ....

3. Place of verbatim : ....

4. Situation : ....

5. Objectives : ....

....

....

....

....

....

....

....

Person	Verbal response	Nonverbal response	Inference

Contd...

Person	Verbal response	Nonverbal response	Inference

Summary

....

....

....

....

....

....

....

Time and place of next interview: ....

Observation Report on Visit to Electroconvulsive Therapy Room

1. Diagram/Blueprint Showing ECT Room

2. Description of Physical Setup of ECT Room

....

....

....

....

....

....

....

3. Equipment Available/Used in ECT Room

....

....

....

....

4. Medications Used in ECT Room

5. Indications for ECT

6. Contraindications for ECT

....
....
....
....

7. Complications of ECT

....
....
....
....
....
....
....

8. Role of Nurse in ECT

A. Pretreatment

....
....
....
....
....
....

B. During treatment

....

C. Post-treatment

Assisting in ECT-1

1. Identification Data

Name of the patient   : ....

Father/Husband name   : ....

Age   : .... Sex : ....

Ward admitted in   : ....

Diagnosis   : ....

Date of admission   : ....

2. Presenting Chief Complaints

....

....

....

....

....

....

3. Indication for ECT

....

....

....

....

....

....

....

....

4. Type of ECT Given

Unilateral/Bilateral   : ....

Direct/Modified   : ....

5. Pre-medications Given

Sl. no.	Name of the drug	Dose	Route	Action

6. Vital Signs

Vital signs	Pre-ECT	During ECT	Post-ECT
Temperature			
Pulse			
Respiration			
Blood pressure			

7. Specific Observation

A. Before ECT

....

....

....

....

....

B. During ECT

C. After ECT

8. Any complication (Before, during or after ECT)

....
....
....
....

9. Nurse's role

....
....
....
....
....
....
....
....

Assisting in ECT-2

1. Identification Data

Name of the patient : ....

Father/husband name : ....

Age : .... Sex : ....

Ward admitted in : ....

Diagnosis : ....

Date of admission : ....

2. Presenting Chief Complaints

....

....

....

....

....

....

....

....

3. Indication for ECT

....

....

....

....

....

....

....

....

4. Type of ECT Given

Unilateral/Bilateral   : ....

Direct/Modified   : ....

5. Pre-medications Given

Sl. no.	Name of the drug	Dose	Route	Action

6. Vital Signs

Vital signs	Pre-ECT	During ECT	Post-ECT
Temperature			
Pulse			
Respiration			
Blood pressure			

7. Specific Observation

A. Before ECT

....

....

....

....

....

....

B. During ECT

C. After ECT

8. Any complication (Before, during or after ECT)

....

....

....

9. Nurse's role

....

....

....

....

....

....

....

....

Assisting in ECT-3

1. Identification Data

Name of the patient : ....

Father/husband name : ....

Age : .... Sex : ....

Ward admitted in : ....

Diagnosis : ....

Date of admission : ....

2. Presenting Chief Complaints

....

....

....

....

....

....

....

3. Indication for ECT

....

....

....

....

....

....

....

....

4. Type of ECT Given

Unilateral/Bilateral   : ....

Direct/Modified   : ....

5. Pre-medications Given

Sl. no.	Name of the drug	Dose	Route	Action

6. Vital Signs

Vital signs	Pre-ECT	During ECT	Post-ECT
Temperature			
Pulse			
Respiration			
Blood pressure			

7. Specific Observation

A. Before ECT

....

....

....

....

....

....

B. During ECT

C. After ECT

8. Any complication (Before, during or after ECT)

9. Nurse's role

Assisting in ECT-4

1. Identification Data

Name of the patient : ....

Father/husband name : ....

Age : .... Sex : ....

Ward admitted in : ....

Diagnosis : ....

Date of admission : ....

2. Presenting Chief Complaints

....

....

....

....

....

....

....

3. Indication for ECT

....

....

....

....

....

....

....

....

4. Type of ECT Given

Unilateral/Bilateral : ....

Direct/Modified   : ....

5. Pre-medications Given

Sl. no.	Name of the drug	Dose	Route	Action

6. Vital Signs

Vital signs	Pre-ECT	During ECT	Post-ECT
Temperature			
Pulse			
Respiration			
Blood pressure			

7. Specific Observation

A. Before ECT

....

....

....

....

....

B. During ECT

C. After ECT

8. Any complication (Before, during or after ECT)

9. Nurse's role

Assisting in ECT-5

1. Identification Data

Name of the patient : ....

Father/husband name : ....

Age : .... Sex : ....

Ward admitted in : ....

Diagnosis : ....

Date of admission : ....

2. Presenting Chief Complaints

....

....

....

....

....

....

....

3. Indication for ECT

....

....

....

....

....

....

....

4. Type of ECT Given

Unilateral/Bilateral : ....

Direct/Modified   : ....

5. Pre-medications Given

Sl. no.	Name of the drug	Dose	Route	Action

6. Vital Signs

Vital signs	Pre-ECT	During ECT	Post-ECT
Temperature			
Pulse			
Respiration			
Blood pressure			

7. Specific Observation

A. Before ECT

....

....

....

....

....

B. During ECT

C. After ECT

8. Any complication (Before, during or after ECT)

9. Nurse's role

Assignment on Psychotherapies-1

Therapy:

1. Meaning and definition

2. Brief description of the therapy

3. Uses

4. Role of a nurse in the therapy

5. Summary

Assignment on Psychotherapies-2

Therapy:

1. Meaning and definition

....
....
....
....
....
....
....

2. Brief description of the therapy

....
....
....
....
....
....
....

3. Uses

....
....
....
....

4. Role of a nurse in the therapy

5. Summary

Assignment on Psychotherapies-3

Therapy:

1. Meaning and definition

2. Brief description of the therapy

3. Uses

4. Role of a nurse in the therapy

5. Summary

....

....

....

....

Assignment on Psychotherapies-4

Therapy:

1. Meaning and definition

....
....
....
....
....
....
....

2. Brief description of the therapy

....
....
....
....
....
....
....
....

3. Uses

....
....
....

4. Role of a nurse in the therapy

5. Summary

Assignment on Psychotherapies-5

Therapy:

1. Meaning and definition

....

....

....

....

....

....

....

2. Brief description of the therapy

....

....

....

....

....

....

....

3. Uses

....

....

....

4. Role of a nurse in the therapy

5. Summary

Drug Study-1

Antipsychotic

1. Name of the Drug : ....

2. Pharmacological Name : ....

3. Mechanism of Action : ....

....

....

....

....

4. Dosage : ....

5. Available Forms : ....

6. Routes of Administration : ....

7. Uses/Indications : ....

....

....

....

8. Contraindications : ....

....

....

....

....

9. Adverse Effects :..

....

....

....

....

....

....

....

10. Nurse's Responsibility :..

....

....

....

....

....

....

....

....

....

....

....

....

Drug Study-2

Antidepressant

1. Name of the Drug : ....

2. Pharmacological Name : ....

3. Mechanism of Action : ....

....

....

....

....

4. Dosage : ....

5. Available Forms : ....

6. Routes of Administration : ....

7. Uses/Indications : ....

....

....

....

....

8. Contraindications : ....

....

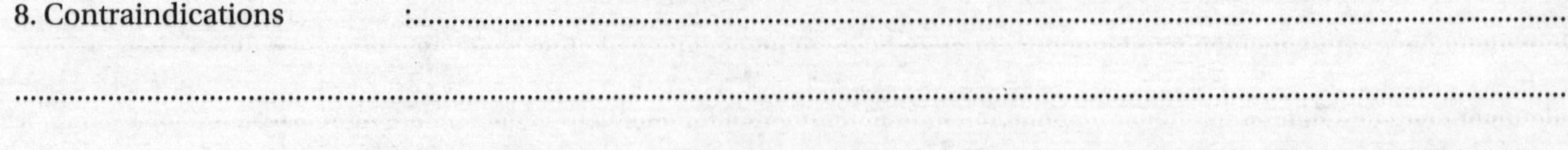

....

....

....

9. Adverse Effects : ....

....

....

....

....

....

....

....

....

10. Nurses' Responsibility : ....

....

....

....

....

....

....

....

....

....

....

....

....

Drug Study-3

Mood Stabilizing Agent

1. Name of the Drug : ....

2. Pharmacological Name : ....

3. Mechanism of Action : ....

....

....

....

....

4. Dosage : ....

5. Available Forms : ....

6. Routes of Administration : ....

7. Uses/Indications : ....

....

....

....

....

8. Contraindications : ....

....

....

....

....

....

9. Adverse Effects :..

....

....

....

....

....

....

....

....

....

10. Nurses' Responsibility :..

....

....

....

....

....

....

....

....

....

....

....

....

....

Drug Study-4

Disulfiram

1. Name of the Drug : ....

2. Pharmacological Name : ....

3. Mechanism of Action : ....

....

....

....

....

....

4. Dosage : ....

5. Available Forms : ....

6. Routes of Administration : ....

7. Uses/Indications : ....

....

....

....

....

....

8. Contraindications : ....

....

....

....

....

9. Adverse Effects :..

....

....

....

....

....

....

....

10. Nurses' Responsibility :..

....

....

....

....

....

....

....

....

....

....

....

....

Drug Study-5

Sedatives

1. Name of the Drug : ....

2. Pharmacological Name : ....

3. Mechanism of Action : ....

....

....

....

....

4. Dosage : ....

5. Available Forms : ....

6. Routes of Administration : ....

7. Uses/Indications : ....

....

....

....

....

8. Contraindications : ....

....

....

....

....

....

9. Adverse Effects : ....

10. Nurses' Responsibility : ....

Drug Study-6

Antiparkinsonian Agent

1. Name of the Drug : ....

2. Pharmacological Name : ....

3. Mechanism of Action : ....

....

....

....

....

4. Dosage : ....

5. Available Forms : ....

6. Routes of Administration : ....

7. Uses/Indications : ....

....

....

....

....

8. Contraindications : ....

....

....

....

9. Adverse Effects :...

10. Nurse's Responsibility :...

Drug Study-7

Anticonvulsant

1. Name of the Drug   : ....

2. Pharmacological Name   : ....

3. Mechanism of Action   : ....

....

....

....

....

....

4. Dosage   : ....

5. Available Forms   : ....

6. Routes of Administration   : ....

7. Uses/Indications   : ....

....

....

....

....

....

8. Contraindications   : ....

....

....

....

....

....

9. Adverse Effects :..

....

....

....

....

....

....

....

10. Nurses' Responsibility :..

....

....

....

....

....

....

....

....

....

....

....

....

Drug Study-8

Anxiolytic

1. Name of the Drug : ....

2. Pharmacological Name : ....

3. Mechanism of Action : ....

....

....

....

....

4. Dosage : ....

5. Available Forms : ....

6. Routes of Administration : ....

7. Uses/Indications : ....

....

....

....

....

8. Contraindications : ....

....

....

....

....

9. Adverse Effects : ....

....

....

....

10. Nurses' Responsibility :

Drug Study-9

Anticraving Agent

1. Name of the Drug : ....

2. Pharmacological Name : ....

3. Mechanism of Action : ....

....

....

....

....

....

4. Dosage : ....

5. Available Forms : ....

6. Routes of Administration : ....

7. Uses/Indications : ....

....

....

....

....

8. Contraindications : ....

....

....

....

9. Adverse Effects   : ....

10. Nurses' Responsibility : ....

Drug Study-10

Other___________________

1. Name of the Drug   : ....

2. Pharmacological Name   : ....

3. Mechanism of Action   : ....

....

....

....

....

4. Dosage   : ....

5. Available Forms   : ....

6. Routes of Administration : ....

7. Uses/Indications   : ....

....

....

....

....

8. Contraindications   : ....

....

....

....

....

9. Adverse Effects   : ....

10. Nurses' Responsibility :

Health Education-1

1. Individual

Name of the patient : ....

Topic : ....

Name of the patient : ....

Age/Sex : ....

Education : ....

Diagnosis of the patient : ....

Method of teaching : ....

Medium of teaching : ....

Audio-visual aids : ....

Duration : ....

Venue : ....

Date : ....

1. General objectives

....

....

....

....

....

....

....

2. Specific objectives

Time	Specific Objectives	Contents	Activities		A-V aids	Method of evaluation
			Teacher	Clients		

Time	Specific Objectives	Contents	Activities		A-V aids	Method of evaluation
			Teacher	Clients		

Contd...

Time	Specific Objectives	Contents	Activities		A-V aids	Method of evaluation
			Teacher	Clients		

Health Education-2

2. Group

Topic   : ....
Group   : ....
Size of the group   : ....
Method of teaching   : ....
Medium of teaching   : ....
Audio-visual aids   : ....
Duration   : ....
Venue   : ....
Date   : ....

1. General objectives

....

....

....

....

....

....

....

2. Specific objectives

....

....

....

....

....

....

....

....

Time	Specific Objectives	Contents	Activities		A-V aids	Method of evaluation
			Teacher	Clients		

Contd...

Time	Specific Objectives	Contents	Activities		A-V aids	Method of evaluation
			Teacher	Clients		

Contd...

Time	Specific Objectives	Contents	Activities		A-V aids	Method of evaluation
			Teacher	Clients		

Community Psychiatry and De-addiction Center

Psychiatric Care Study on Drug Dependency

1. Identification Data

Name of the patient : ....

Father/Husband name : ....

Age : ....Sex: ....

Ward admitted in : ....

Diagnosis : ....

Date of admission : ....

Marital status : ....

Religion : ....

Nationality : ....

Educational status : ....

Occupation : ....

Family income/month : ....

Mode of admission : .... Voluntary/Brought by Relatives/Through court/Through police

2. Informant

Name of the informant : ....

Relation with patient : ....

Duration of stay with patient: ....

3. Presenting Chief Complaints

....

....

....

....

....

....

....

....

4. History of Present Illness
(Duration, mode of onset, course of illness, intensity, precipitating factors, associated disturbances, etc.)

....

....

....

....

....

....

....

5. Past Psychiatric History
(Past psychiatric problems, hospitalization, treatment history, previous episode of presenting complaints)

....

....

....

....

....

....

....

6. Past Medical History
(Past medical problems, hospitalization, treatment history, surgery, if any, etc.)

....

....

....

....

....

....

....

7. Family History

Type of family: Nuclear/Joint

Brief description of family: (Parents, siblings, spouse, children)

....

....

....

....

....

....

....

Family psychiatric history

(Behavioral/Emotional problems in any family member, drugs/Alcohol abuse in family, etc.)

....

....

....

....

....

....

....

....

8. Personal History (Only significant in brief)

....

....

....

....

....

....

....

9. Mental Status Examination (Significant findings in brief)

A. General appearance and behavior

....

....

....

....

....

....

....

B. Speech

....

....

....

....

....

....

C. Mood and affect

Subjective mood : ....

Objective mood (affect) : ....

....

....

....

....

....

....

D. Thought

....

....

....

....

....

....

E. Perception

....
....
....
....
....
....
....
....

F. Cognitive functions

i. Consciousness : .... Conscious/Cloudy/Comatose

ii. Orientation

- Time : ....Oriented/Disoriented
- Place : ....Oriented/Disoriented
- Person : ....Oriented/Disoriented

iii. Attention and concentration

- Arousal : .... Normal/Difficulty
- Attention : ....Intact/Altered
- Concentration : ....Intact/Altered

iv. Memory

- Immediate : ....Intact/Altered
- Recent : ....Intact/Altered
- Remote : ....Intact/Altered

v. Intelligence

- General information : ....Intact/Altered
- Arithmetic ability : ....Intact/Altered

vi. Abstraction

- Interpretation of proverbs : ....
- Similarities between paired objects : ....
- Dissimilarities between paired objects: ....
- Abstraction : Intact/Altered

vii. Judgment

- Personal : .... Intact/Impaired

- ◆ Social : .... Intact/Impaired
- ◆ Test : .... Intact/Impaired

G. Insight

- Awareness of abnormal behavior: .... Yes/No/Maybe
- Attribution to physical cause : .... Yes/No/Maybe
- Willingness to take treatment : .... Yes/No/Maybe

10. Physical examination (Significant findings)

A. Anthropometric measurements

- Height : ....
- Weight : ....
- Head circumference : ....
- Chest circumference : ....
- Mid-arm circumference : ....

B. General appearance

....

....

....

....

....

....

C. Head-to-toe examination (Significant findings, if any)

....

....

....

....

....

....

....

11. Investigations

Sl. no.	Investigation	Normal value	Patient's value	Inference

12. Medical Treatment

Sl. no.	Drug	Action	Dose	Frequency	Route

Sl. no.	Drug	Action	Dose	Frequency	Route

13. ECT (If any)

....

....

....

....

....

....

....

14. Psychological Therapy (If any)

....

....

....

....

....

....

....

....

15. Comparison Between Patient and Book Picture

Definition of disease

Patient picture	Book picture
Clinical features	
Psychopathology	

Contd...

Diagnostic evaluation	
Management	
Prognosis	

16. List of Nursing Diagnosis

....
....
....
....

17. Nursing Care Plan

Nursing diagnosis:

Goal/Expected outcome

Assessment	Intervention	Implementation	Evaluation

Nursing diagnosis:

Goal/Expected outcome

Assessment	Intervention	Implementation	Evaluation

Nursing diagnosis:

Goal/Expected outcome

Assessment	Intervention	Implementation	Evaluation

Nursing diagnosis:

Goal/Expected outcome

Assessment	Intervention	Implementation	Evaluation

18. Health Education

19. Conclusion

Observation Report on Visit to De-addiction Center

1. Introduction of the de-addiction centre

....

....

....

....

....

....

....

2. Physical setup of the de-addiction centre

....

....

....

....

....

....

....

3. Objectives of the de-addiction centre

....

....

....

....

4. Functions of the de-addiction centre

5. Staff of the de-addiction centre

6. Summary of the visit

....
....
....
....

Observation Report on Visit to Rehabilitation Center

1. Introduction of the rehabilitation centre

2. Physical setup of the rehabilitation centre

3. Objectives of the rehabilitation centre

....

....

....

4. Functions of the rehabilitation centre

....

....

....

....

....

....

....

....

5. Staff of the rehabilitation centre

....

....

....

....

....

....

....

....

6. Summary of the visit

....

....

....

....

....

....

....

....

Bibliography

1. Basavanthappa BT. Community Health Nursing, 1st ed. 1999, Jaypee Brothers, New Delhi.

2. Kapoor Bimla. Text Book of Psychiatric Nursing, Vol II, 1st ed. Kumar Publishing House, New Delhi.

3. Neeraja KP. Essentials of Mental Health and Psychiatric Nursing, Vol II, 2nd ed. Jaypee Brothers, New Delhi.

4. Sreevani R. A Guide to Mental Health and Psychiatric Nursing, 1st ed. 2004, Jaypee Brothers, New Delhi.

5. Stuart and Laraia. Principles and Practice of Psychiatric Nursing, 8th ed. 2005, Elsevier Publication.

6. http://www.nandanursingdiagnosislist.org/psychosocial-nursing-diagnosis.